LG. PRINT
616.722   Kantrowitz,Fred G.
KAN   Taking control of
          of arthritis

NOV 23 1997

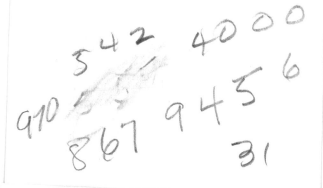

"BOOKS MAY BE
RENEWED BY PHONE"

FORT MORGAN PUBLIC LIBRARY
414 MAIN STREET
FORT MORGAN, CO 80701
867-9456

GAYLORD M

TAKING CONTROL OF
ARTHRITIS

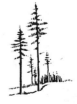

5+5 9/97 21.95

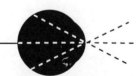

**This Large Print Book carries the
Seal of Approval of N.A.V.H.**

TAKING CONTROL OF
ARTHRITIS

Property of:
Fort Morgan Public Library
414 Main Street
Fort Morgan, Colorado

Fred G. Kantrowitz, M.D.

Thorndike Press • Thorndike, Maine

Library of Congress Cataloging in Publication Data:

Kantrowitz, Fred G.
  Taking control of arthritis / Fred G. Kantrowitz.
    p. cm.
  Includes index.
  ISBN 1-56054-235-7 (alk. paper : lg. print)
  ISBN 1-56054-957-2 (alk. paper : lg. print : pbk.)
  1. Arthritis—Popular works. 2. Large type books.
I. Title. II. Title: Arthritis.
  [RC933.K36   1991]   91-22638
  616.7'22—dc20   CIP

Copyright © 1990 by Fred G. Kantrowitz, M.D.
All rights reserved.

Thorndike Press Large Print edition published in 1991
by arrangement with HarperCollins Publishers.

Cover design by Ralph Lizotte.

The tree indicium is a trademark of Thorndike Press.

This book is printed on acid-free, high opacity paper.

To Anne, Gregory, and William.
No man could ask for more.

Contents

Acknowledgments

This book is a labor of love that could not have been accomplished without the support of numerous people.

I want to thank Susan Manfred and Charles Shepherd of the Arthritis Foundation, Donna Cosola of the American College of Rheumatology, and Jane Bruckel of the Ankylosing Spondylitis Association for their help and suggestions. Nancy and Betsy for organizing my professional life. Eamon Dolan of Harper-Collins for his perceptions and enthusiasm. Joanne and Rick, so far but yet so close — hard work does indeed pay off. Special thanks to the celebrities who graciously consented to be interviewed and whose triumphs over arthritis will serve as an inspiration to the reader. A big thank you to my patients — the people who asked the questions in this book. And, finally, to Theo and Diane, who were always there when I needed them.

The opinions expressed in this book are my own and are not a substitute for conventional medical care. All questions should be directed to your doctor. Do not use this book to self-diagnose, treat, or determine side effects of therapy. Consult your physician and other appropriate health care professionals before beginning any new treatment program, including diet and exercise.

1

The Problem

If you have been fortunate enough to see dancer Juliet Prowse perform, you probably came away with the impression that she is quite an entertainer. You marveled at her stamina, her grace, but mostly at her physical presence. Few dancers can kick their legs higher than Juliet Prowse.

Perhaps you saw her in Las Vegas, where she performed regularly for over twenty-five years. Or maybe it was in hits such as *Irma La Douce, On a Clear Day, You Can See Forever,* or *Mame.* Perhaps it was in London, where she starred in a record-breaking run of *Sweet Charity.*

If you have seen Juliet Prowse perform, it will probably surprise you to hear she has arthritis. Maybe, on second thought, you will think about it for a bit, remember that she's over 50 years old, and say it is not so surprising after all. But Juliet Prowse has had arthritis for over twenty-five years — in other words, for most of her career.

She is living testimony that arthritis is a

disease that can be treated, and treated effectively. You don't have to live with it; it does not have to dominate your life.

Unfortunately, Juliet Prowse's experience does not always represent the norm. In contrast, consider the following words uttered by Edna Smith, a 64-year-old woman with rheumatoid arthritis. They are all too familiar.

"When you have arthritis no one wants to do anything for you — so you give up."

Edna Smith's disease started when she was 18 years old. She saw scores of physicians. No one encouraged her. In her own words, no one helped her.

How typical is Edna Smith's story? How big a problem is arthritis? Over thirty-seven million Americans have arthritis. The average patient with rheumatoid or osteoarthritis, the two most common types, is significantly handicapped for one out of every four weeks and spends almost one and one half days per month in bed. Among students and working patients, two and one half work days per month are lost; thirty percent can't work at all. The economic impact of arthritis is staggering. Medical costs and lost wages account for billions of dollars a year.

Probably no other disease results in so much suffering, in so many people, for such a prolonged period of time. "At least it doesn't kill you," some skeptics would say. Wrong. It does, and in many ways.

It surprises many people to discover that there are over a hundred different types of arthritis. As you have already seen, it is not restricted to the elderly. Many types are commonly seen in young people. Some are exclusively diseases of youth.

Osteoarthritis is a wear-and-tear process most often observed in older individuals. As longevity is increasing, the percentage of the elderly in the population is increasing as well, thus adding to the ranks of people suffering from this problem. Even osteoarthritis is not restricted to senior citizens, however. As Americans have become aware of the importance of keeping fit, we have engaged in a ballooning number of physical activities — jogging, aerobics, swimming, and tennis, to list but a few. As a result, greater numbers of people are at risk to develop athletic injuries. Many will develop arthritis in previously injured joints. It is sometimes difficult to distinguish the knees of a 30-year-old basketball player from those of people in their 70s or 80s. In fact, the basketball player's knees are often in worse shape!

Given the above, is Edna Smith's experience unusual? One might think physicians would be expert at diagnosing and treating arthritic conditions. After all, Americans visit doctors millions of times a year to have their arthritis evaluated and treated. But a number of objective criteria indicate that arthritis is one of the most poorly treated diseases.

Why is this? In part it is because of how we train our doctors. Physicians are trained in hospitals, where for the most part they take care of patients with acute, life-threatening illnesses. This is more true now than ever because of the trend to treat people on an outpatient basis whenever possible. Since few patients with arthritis are admitted to hospitals for treatment of their joint problems, trainees are underexposed to this set of medical problems.

Although patients with arthritis are seen in hospital outpatient departments, most trainees attend only one such clinic a week. Thankfully, this is beginning to change, and many teaching hospitals are beginning to emphasize the importance of outpatient medicine.

Still, it is not unusual for a physician to graduate from a highly renowned training program without having taken care of one patient with rheumatoid arthritis. There are over 2.5 million people in the United States with this illness, so it is a common disease, yet some trainees are more likely to take care of patients with rare illnesses (which they will probably never see in their practices) than common arthritic conditions.

Fortunately the situation is not as discouraging as it may sound. Once physicians get into the real world they realize the scope of the problem. By applying their theoretical knowledge, they learn on the job and ultimately take adequate care of their patients with arthritis.

But things don't always work out well, at least in part because of our attitudes toward arthritis. Since arthritis is frequently perceived as a disease for which little can be done, patients often don't pressure their doctors to make them better. As a result they are frequently told they have to live with their problem. Pain medications are prescribed. Some patients become dependent on drugs, prescription and otherwise, or alcohol, and that's wrong, because there's a lot that can be done to treat arthritis. But in order to assure yourself of the best medicine has to offer, you have to take control of your problem. You have to learn what arthritis is and how it can be helped.

Help means more than taking pills, although that may be very important. It means being as healthy as you can be. It means knowing when to exercise and when not to exercise. It means knowing about diet, sleep, stress, interpersonal relations, and a lot of other important things that may not appear to have a lot to do with bones and joints.

There are physicians who specialize in the treatment of arthritic conditions, whose help you may or may not need. Rheumatologists spend three years in an accredited internal medicine training program, then two additional years in a rheumatology fellowship. They must pass national board exams in internal medicine and rheumatology in order to become board-certified rheumatologists, of which there are approximately 2500 in the United States. Most rheumatologists in this country belong to a professional organization called the American College of Rheumatology.

There is a national organization devoted to supporting research to find the cure for arthritis and to improve the quality of life for patients affected by arthritis. The Arthritis Foundation is a voluntary, nonprofit organization with chapters in almost every state. In addition to promoting research, it supports professional and community education, various services for people with arthritis, and serves as an advocate on legislative issues. A number of similar national organizations are devoted to specific types of arthritis.

So there's a lot of help available and a lot to learn. Despite this, patients with arthritis are often frustrated as their concerns are not addressed, their questions left unanswered. It is striking how often the same questions are asked and the same prejudices unmasked because the same myths have been perpetuated. The same fears, initially unspoken, ultimately surface.

The following chapters — dealing with the most commonly asked questions about arthritis — address these issues. The questions range from the obvious to the subtle, the theoretical to the practical, in some cases from the ridiculous to the sublime. But they all have one thing in common — they have been asked by real people with real concerns, and as such they deserve to be answered. Only then will you be able to take control of your arthritis.

2

The Most Asked Question: Aren't I Too Young to Get Arthritis?

One of the major medical misconceptions in our society is that arthritis is exclusively a disease of the elderly. Another is that we're supposed to have aches and pains as we grow older, that it's simply part of the aging process. Perpetuation of these myths would be unimportant but for one crucial factor — arthritis can be treated, and in many cases rather easily. So if you labor under the misconception that you're too young to have arthritis, or you think you're supposed to feel stiff just because you're 50 or 60 or 70 years old, you may be doing yourself a disservice.

These attitudes are reflected in the following quotes.

"I thought only old people got arthritis."
— LYNN ADAMS,
WOMEN'S PROFESSIONAL
RACQUETBALL CHAMPION

"I didn't know I had arthritis. I thought I was getting old."
— MICKEY MANTLE,
RETIRED BASEBALL SUPERSTAR

"I'm not old enough, Doc. You've got to be wrong. I can't have arthritis."
— KEVIN CALLAHAN,
A 76-YEAR-OLD RETIRED POLICEMAN — PROVING THAT EVERYTHING IS RELATIVE.

Lynn Adams is the world's premier female racquetball player. Since the creation of the Women's Professional Racquetball Association in 1979, she has won six national championships and more matches, titles, and money than any other player. Now in her early 30s, Ms. Adams is the picture of athletic perfection on the racquetball court. Yet she has had rheumatoid arthritis since she was just 16 years old.

She'll never forget how it started. Upon awakening one morning she discovered that her wrist was swollen and immobile. It was so painful she thought it was broken and went to a local emergency room, where an x-ray proved negative. Told she had a virus, she was reassured when the pain went away within the next three days. But a week later the same

19

thing happened in her knee, and soon other joints were involved. Within a month, the diagnosis was made — rheumatoid arthritis.

Incredulous at first, she and her family ultimately accepted her fate. Yet it wasn't until the age of 21 that "it dawned on me I was going to have this for the rest of my life."

Through enlightened medical care ("I had a progressive doctor"), which encouraged her to lead as active a life as possible, a thirst for knowledge regarding her problem, and adherence to sound principles of health care, Ms. Adams has taken control of her illness and gone on to become a world-class athlete. You'll find more on how she did this in the chapters to come.

Having grown up in New York, I have vivid memories of the local sports heroes, one of the most prominent of whom was Mickey Mantle. Of those recollections, none is more clear than the time Mantle hit a home run that almost went out of Yankee Stadium, a feat never accomplished, not even by Babe Ruth. It missed by a mere foot. Barely 12 years old at the time, I sat transfixed in front of the television as Mantle rounded the bases, marveling at the power of one of the greatest home run hitters in the history of the game.

Little did I know I would be interviewing Mantle some thirty years later, his life indelibly altered by the illness I have devoted my professional career to treating.

It all started in 1951, Mantle's rookie year, a year that shaped his entire career and ultimately his retirement from baseball. In the World Series, the Yankees played the Giants. Mantle was in right field. Another all-time great, Joe DiMaggio, was playing center field. Ironically, DiMaggio was suffering from an arthritic problem of his own, heel spurs, which had considerably reduced his mobility. So Casey Stengel, the Yankee manager, instructed Mantle to take as many balls hit toward center as he could, fearing DiMaggio would not be able to cover the necessary territory.

Willie Mays, also in his first year, hit a fly ball toward short right center field. Remembering Stengel's orders, Mantle bolted toward the ball, abruptly stopping when he heard DiMaggio yell, "I got it." Mantle's spikes caught on the cover of a drain pipe buried in the outfield grass, and he collapsed in pain, tearing the ligaments in his right knee.

He was operated on a few days later and returned home to Commerce, Oklahoma, for the off-season. When the cast was removed, he skipped his rehabilitation exercises. He thought the muscles would automatically strengthen — after all, he was 20 years old and, in his words, thought he was Superman. It was one of the biggest mistakes he ever made.

He played the rest of his career in pain. His right knee never fully recovered. Trying to compensate, he put extra weight on his left knee, ultimately damaging it as well. By spring training of 1969 he couldn't even do jumping jacks and realized it was time to retire. He called it "the saddest day of my life." Four more knee operations followed, but the pain continued. He reached the point where he couldn't play golf, his main form of exercise and recreation. He could barely climb stairs. When asked about his reaction to giving up golf, he said, "I reached a point where I didn't worry about golf. I thought I wasn't going to be able to get around at all."

Despite his constant knee pain, he said, "I didn't know I had arthritis. I thought I was getting old." Like many Americans, Mantle did not equate his increasing infirmity with arthritis but with his age. In fact, it wasn't until 1987 that Mantle discovered he had osteoarthritis.

Age is relative. Kevin Callahan was referred to me after his family complained to his primary care doctor that he was having difficulty walking and using his hands. After examining him, I was convinced Mr. Callahan had rheumatoid arthritis. The joints characteristically involved in rheumatoid arthritis were all warm, red, and swollen, and I didn't entertain any other diagnosis. I was confused, however, because he did not have any complaints — it was his family who thought there was a problem. I pressed the issue, but the retired policeman was steadfast. Nothing bothered him.

Despite his lack of complaints I suggested treatment with an anti-inflammatory medication, and after much cajoling by his family he reluctantly agreed. When he returned for his next appointment I immediately noted the change. His sad, droopy face was replaced by twinkling eyes and a broad smile. "You wouldn't believe how much better I feel," he said. "I thought I was supposed to feel that way when I was seventy-six." When I told him it wasn't his age but his arthritis, he was surprised, stating he was too young to have arthritis!

Arthritis is frequently an insidious process, an illness whose effects may be felt only gradually. We think of most illnesses as events that have specific beginnings, yet the birth of arthritis can be so subtle it is barely noticed. No wonder it is often confused with aging. We underestimate the presence of arthritis throughout the age spectrum. Lynn Adams thought she was too young at 16. Mickey Mantle thought he was supposed to feel pain because he was getting older. Kevin Callahan's difficulties developed so insidiously he thought he was "supposed to feel that way." Indeed, many forms of arthritis are more common in young and middle-aged adults than in the elderly. Some types are almost completely restricted to children. But with a few minor exceptions, no type is restricted to the elderly.

When I first decided to become a rheumatologist, my classmates warned me I would be dealing exclusively with older individuals. Although they knew I enjoyed working with the elderly, they thought a "mix" of patients would be more interesting. Ironically, if they were to see my waiting room they'd see that mix, a true cross-section of America — young and old, male and female. Doctors and medical students aren't immune to myths and misconceptions.

Many of the people whose histories are described in this book developed their arthritis at relatively early ages. Jack Kramer is one of the legends of American tennis; he was forced to retire in his early 30s because of arthritis in his back. Five-time Wimbledon champ Vic Seixas, who played on more Davis

Cup teams than any other American tennis player, developed arthritis in his knees in his late 50s — perhaps a more "traditional" age to develop the disease, but relatively young by our societal standards nevertheless. Bobby Orr, one of the greatest professional hockey players, had developed arthritis by the time he was 30.

The development of arthritis at an "early" age is hardly restricted to competitive athletes. Actress Jane Withers, a child star by the age of 8, gained fame and fortune by appearing in films with Shirley Temple and Mickey Rooney but is perhaps better known as Josephine, the lady plumber, from a long-running TV commercial. Ms. Withers developed rheumatoid arthritis at the age of 27. Dancer Donna McKechnie, the original star of *A Chorus Line,* developed rheumatoid arthritis at the age of 36. These are typical ages for the development of this disease. Dancer Juliet Prowse was told she had arthritis when she was in her early 20s. Actress Annie Potts developed arthritis as a result of an automobile accident when she was 21. The French Impressionist painter Renoir was stricken with rheumatoid arthritis at the age of 56 — yet some of his best painting was still to come. John F. Kennedy was a young man when he first developed back problems. Some of the most famous pictures of the Kennedy White House feature the President's favorite rocking chair, a solace for his aches and pains.

So if you experience an ache here, a pain there, it may be the beginning of arthritis — no matter what your age. On the other hand, every time a joint hurts it doesn't mean you have arthritis. The following chapters describe what arthritis is, how the diagnosis is made, and how it is treated — both by you and your doctor.

3

The Basics

Learn the ABC of science before you
try to ascend to its summit.
— IVAN PETROVICH PAVLOV

Every building starts with a foundation.
Without a strong foundation, the floors
that rise above it are insecure, ready to
topple at a moment's notice. Similarly, in
order to fully understand the concepts
that follow, we must start with the basics,
the simplest definitions and principles.

So we start with the most fundamental
of all questions.

What is arthritis?

The word *arthritis* is derived from the
Greek and literally means "inflammation
of a joint." *Inflammation* classically consists of redness, pain, heat, and swelling.
The term is often confusing, however, because all four of these ele-ments may not
appear concurrently — more on this in

where two bones are joined, usually so they can move. Anatomically, there are three types of joints:

1. *Synarthrodial* — joints that, surprisingly, are immobile (note the above definition; joints usually — but not always — move). An example of this type of joint occurs in the skull, which is not a single large bone but consists of a number of smaller bones. These bones meet at so-called suture joints.

2. *Amphiarthrodial* — joints that are slightly movable. These joints are of special interest because many of them are not thought of as joints, yet they often become arthritic. For example, the spine consists of a number of bones called vertebral bodies; they are joined at facet joints. The pelvis, like the skull, consists of a number of bones. Those bones come together in the back at the sacroiliac joint, another joint that can become arthritic. There are a number of other slightly movable joints, many of which are the source of unsuspected arthritic pain. They will be identified as we proceed.

3. *Diarthrodial* — joints that are freely movable. These are the "obvious" joints such as the knee and the hip. Diarthrodial joints con-

sist of a number of different structures. The ends of the two bones forming the joint are covered by a firm, elastic material called *cartilage,* which is also present in some slightly movable joints. The cartilage provides a smooth surface, thereby facilitating motion. Thus, in most joints, cartilage rubs against cartilage, not bone against bone. *Ligaments* hold the bones in a joint together, and *tendons* attach muscles to bones. The latter are analogous to cables. The above structures are surrounded by a *capsule,* the inside of which is lined by a material called *synovial tissue* or the *synovial membrane.* This tissue produces antibodies, which protect the joint, as well as fluid, which bathes and lubricates the joint. Thus it is normal for joints to contain a small amount of fluid. The presence of excess fluid ("water on the knee") is abnormal.

There are more joints in the body than one would think, and all movable and slightly movable joints are capable of becoming inflamed. For example, that backache you've attributed to muscle spasm could very well be arthritic in nature.

In general, arthritis is divided into two broad categories — inflammatory and degenerative, or mechanical. This terminology can be confusing because inflammation may be present in degenerative types of arthritis although it is usually minor.

In inflammatory illnesses such as rheumatoid arthritis, the inflammation begins in the synovial membrane and then spreads, potentially destroying the cartilage and underlying bone.

Degenerative arthritis, also called osteoarthritis, is a wear-and-tear process. It is primarily a disease of cartilage, which initially softens, cracks, and then loses its elasticity. It wears away to varying degrees. In some instances it is totally destroyed, leaving the ends of the bones devoid of its protective effects. As the normal smooth surface of the cartilage is destroyed, it becomes difficult and painful to move the joint. Destructive changes in the underlying bone often follow, and the joint begins to lose its normal shape. The ends of the bones thicken and form bony growths in response to the increased stress. These growths are called *spurs* and usually occur where the ligaments attach to the bone. Small pieces of cartilage or bone sometimes chip off into the joint space. These in turn may irritate the joint, leading to inflammation. All of these changes contribute to the pain associated with osteoarthritis.

It takes time for osteoarthritis to develop. The older you are, the more likely you are to develop osteoarthritis. It is present to some degree in virtually everyone over the age of 65, but relatively few people develop significant symptoms.

What are the most common causes of osteoarthritis?

Although we aren't sure about the causes of osteoarthritis, there are a number of theories, as follows.

• *Heredity*. Joints appear to "wear out" more easily in some people than in others. This may be because their cartilage is "softer" than normal or because there are subtle defects in the structure of their joints. Over time this results in one area of cartilage being stressed more than others, and the cartilage eventually succumbs to the increased pressure.

The knowledge that arthritis can be hereditary was what drove dancer and actress Cyd Charisse to seek medical help relatively soon after she developed pain in her hands and began having difficulty opening jars. Her mother was almost crippled by osteoarthritis, so she was not surprised when she developed the same problem. Determined to avoid her mother's fate, she soon embarked upon a program of medication and exercise and has responded beautifully. The costar of hit films such as *Singin' in the Rain, The Band Wagon,* and *Brigadoon,* Cyd Charisse is one of the few Hollywood leading ladies who has danced with both Gene Kelly and Fred Astaire. Today she remains as active and vibrant as ever, taking care of her arthritis with the same precision she exhibited in her legendary dance steps.

• *Birth defects* that distort the normal anatomy of the joint can be associated with the ultimate development of arthritis. For example, children born with dislocated hips often develop osteoarthritis.

• *Obesity* appears to correlate with the development of osteoarthritis, especially of the knee. This association is stronger in women than in men.

• *Other forms of arthritis* may damage cartilage, facilitating the development of osteoarthritis. For example, rheumatoid arthritis and osteoarthritis may be found in the same joint.

• *Physical stress.* Occupational overuse of joints and joint injuries subject the cartilage to extra stress and may predispose to the development of osteoarthritis in later life. This type of arthritis is also called *traumatic arthritis* or *traumatic osteoarthritis*. It may occur as a result of an accident, as happened to actress Annie Potts when she was 21. The co-star of the popular TV series "Designing Women" developed arthritis in joints injured in a car accident she was lucky to survive. Her right ankle "hardly works," and she has been told she will eventually need hip surgery. If you closely observe her character, Mary Jo Shively, you will see she occasionally walks with a slight limp. If she is having a particularly rough day, camera angles are situated so she is only seen from the waist up. Although Annie Potts is often in pain, she has never allowed her arthritis to interfere with her career.

Athletic injuries are another prominent cause of traumatic osteoarthritis. At the age of 18 Bobby Orr was a professional hockey player, a defenseman for the Boston Bruins. Considered one of the greatest players ever to lace up a pair of skates, Bobby Orr was out of hockey by the time he was 29 years old. He injured his left knee in 1968, his second professional season. The injury required surgery. He was to undergo an additional ten operations during his career, all on the left knee. He played in pain, much as Mickey Mantle did. By the time he left hockey, Orr already had osteoarthritis in his knee. A good deal of the cartilage is now gone. The motion is a bit restricted and the knee aches intermittently. He can't run, but he still stays in shape by using exercise machines.

Orr downplays the discomfort and hasn't allowed it to dominate his life. He isn't bitter and wouldn't have changed a thing. As he puts it when describing hockey, "Contact is a big part of the game." Since he was such a dominating player, he handled the puck an inordinate amount of the time, making him a ripe target for opposing players. "I could have played a different game, but I didn't."

Although he found the going a bit rough when he first retired, he has done extremely well. Friendly, cooperative, and modest, he is now as successful out of hockey as he was in it. As he said, tongue in cheek, "Things are going great in the business world — at least you don't get beat up."

Former Baltimore Colt quarterback Johnny Unitas's story is a bit more typical in that most of his arthritis developed after the conclusion of his illustrious career. He retired in 1973 at the age of 40, and osteoarthritis gradually developed in joints injured numerous times during his playing days. Many of his finger joints are swollen. Osteoarthritis in his knees prevents him from running. He enjoys a number of activities, such as fishing and golf, that don't put a lot of stress on his knees. Outdoor chores such as cutting grass and chopping wood are a particular passion.

Johnny Unitas has a great attitude, just like Bobby Orr. He doesn't let his arthritis get him down. Upbeat and content, he now devotes the same time and energy to his successful computer company that he did to playing football.

Injuries that lead to arthritis are not restricted to sports such as hockey and football. Dancers are athletes as well.

You have already been introduced to Juliet Prowse. She was born in India, and her family moved to South Africa after her father's untimely death. She began studying ballet at the age of 6. By the time she was 12 her instructors realized she was something special. By the age of 14 she was dancing every day, and she moved to London for advanced training at the age of 17.

Ultimately told she was too tall for ballet, she redirected her efforts to modern dance. It was not long before her talent was recognized. Choreographer Jack Cole signed her for the London production of *Gentlemen Marry Brunettes*. She then joined the London company of *Kismet* stepping into the lead role when the original star was forced to withdraw. She starred in that show for almost two years before forming her own act and appearing in Europe's most prestigious nightclubs. While performing in Spain, she received a cable from producer Hermes Pan. The next thing she knew she was in Hollywood, performing in 20th Century Fox's lavish production of *Can Can*.

By the time she arrived in the United States, Juliet Prowse already had pain in her toes and back. She said, "In the beginning I didn't know what was wrong. I thought it was something to put up with." By her mid-20s, the diagnosis of osteoarthritis was made. It was an intermittent problem until her late 30s, when it intensified.

Most of Juliet Prowse's arthritis occurred in joints she injured while dancing early in her career. Some of those injuries never got a chance to heal. As she put it, "Instead of taking it easy, I intensified my dancing — after all, that was my work."

A word of caution is in order here. Not every athlete develops arthritis, and this should not be construed as a plea to curtail your activities. It is a plea, however, to take care of yourself, to not ignore pain, and to see your doctor as needed. These issues will be discussed as we proceed.

Now that we know what arthritis is, what about the different types? After patients are told they have arthritis, they invariably want to know what kind they have. This is asked in a variety of ways.

What are the major differences between rheumatoid and osteoarthritis?

Rheumatoid arthritis is the most common type of inflammatory arthritis and usually involves many joints. It is a *systemic disease,* which can affect the entire body, including not only the joints but the eyes, heart, lungs, blood vessels, skin, muscles, and nerves. It may cause anemia as well. However, most patients do not develop organ complications, and those who do can usually be helped to a significant degree.

People with rheumatoid arthritis often feel ill, almost as if they have the flu. They may lose weight and tire easily. Fatigue is an underappreciated manifestation of rheumatoid arthritis, often incorrectly attributed to depression — after all, if you have rheumatoid arthritis, you are entitled to be depressed. In addition, rheumatoid arthritis is primarily a disease of young women, a group frequently overdiagnosed as being depressed in the first place. When told the true cause of their fatigue, most patients are extremely relieved and grateful for the explanation. It is indeed comforting to realize that one's complaints are not a product of one's imagination.

Rheumatoid arthritis is a common illness, which affects about one percent of the population, or approximately 2.5 million Americans, with a ratio of approximately three women to one man. It usually begins between the ages of 30 and 50, but spares no age group. One of my patients was 95 years old when he developed the disease.

Osteoarthritis is the prototypical mechanical or degenerative form of arthritis. In fact, it is often called *degenerative joint disease.*

Although osteoarthritis may involve many joints, it usually involves fewer than rheumatoid arthritis. In fact, it may involve only one or two joints, often the knees or hips.

Patients don't feel physically ill, as they often do with rheumatoid arthritis, but if the pain is severe enough they may have other complaints. Pain, no matter what the source, can result in symptoms such as fatigue, depression, irritability, and interruption in normal sleep patterns. These can occur in rheumatoid arthritis as well. Thus, even though osteoarthritis is a joint disease, like rheumatoid arthritis it may result in more global complaints.

What kind do I have — rheumatoid arthritis or osteoarthritis? Do I have the crippling type or the other one?

When patients ask if they have the crippling type of arthritis, I ask which kind they think is capable of doing the most damage. Interestingly, half say osteoarthritis, the other half say rheumatoid arthritis. Patients who have the type they consider crippling are devastated by their diagnosis. If they have the other type, they are relieved.

Although prognosis, or the predicted outcome of a disease, is not the subject of this question, I cannot use the word *crippling* without interjecting a comment. *The vast majority of patients with arthritis do not wind up crippled.* In this age of modern medicine, there are very few people who can't be helped significantly. I have been a rheumatologist for almost fifteen years. During that time, not one of my patients has wound up in a wheelchair. This observation is not offered as an idle boast, but rather reflects our ability to treat patients with arthritis.

So which is the crippling type of arthritis? In the near future, we may be able to say neither one. For the time being, however, both are capable of causing major problems but, when properly treated, usually do not.

When patients are told they don't have either osteoarthritis or rheumatoid arthritis, they are often surprised, not realizing there are indeed other types. The next question usually follows.

What other types of arthritis are there?

There are actually over one hundred conditions that afflict joints. A few of the more common are listed below.

Psoriatic Arthritis

Psoriasis is a common skin condition that causes scaly red patches on various parts of the body. It is estimated to exist in one to two percent of the population; five to eight percent of these individuals have an accompanying arthritis called psoriatic arthritis (further described in Chapter 6). The skin disease may be so minimal that the patient is unaware of it, small patches hiding in the navel, armpits, groin, under the breasts, or

40

behind the elbows being the only evidence of its presence. When it occurs in the scalp it may be confused with simple dandruff. To make matters more complicated, in some cases the arthritis precedes the development of the psoriasis. The nails may also be involved, one of the most common abnormalities being the presence of multiple small pits. Their presence in the absence of skin involvement is often a valuable clue in making the correct diagnosis.

The peak age of onset is between 36 and 45, so this is another type of arthritis that is a "young" person's disease. Particularly severe cases often begin before the age of 20.

The most commonly involved joints are the fingers and toes, but many joints can be affected. Approximately five percent of patients with psoriatic arthritis suffer from arthritis of the spine, which is described below.

Ankylosing Spondylitis

This term is derived from the Greek. *Ankylosing* means "stiff," *spondyl* refers to the spine, and *itis* means "inflammation." It is primarily a disease of the spine, which initially becomes inflamed and in severe cases ultimately becomes fused.

The illness usually begins in the sacroiliac joints, located where two of the bones that form the pelvis, namely the sacrum and iliac, come together. The sacroiliac joints are in the low back, on both sides of the spine, approximately in the area where most people have a dimple, just above the buttocks. Typically, patients with ankylosing spondylitis experience low back pain and stiffness that is unrelieved by rest. Approximately one third of patients have involvement of more "traditional" joints, such as the shoulders, hips, and knees. Almost any joint can be involved. Tendinitis, or inflammation of a tendon, is also a feature of the disease. The tendons around the ankle and feet are commonly involved.

Like rheumatoid arthritis, ankylosing spondylitis is a systemic disease that may involve parts of the body other than joints. Inflammation of the eye is probably the most common complication, occurring in approximately twenty-five percent of patients during the course of their illness. Thus pain or redness in the eye should not simply be dismissed as an irritation, but is an indication to seek medical attention. Heart and lung disease occur less commonly, most often in patients with longstanding disease. Most of the time these complications are of little consequence.

Finally, like those with rheumatoid arthritis, patients with ankylosing spondylitis may suffer from anemia, fatigue, weight loss, and, rarely, even low-grade fevers.

Ankylosing spondylitis is truly a young person's disease, often beginning prior to the age of 20. Approximately five percent of cases begin in childhood. It almost never begins after the age of 40 unless it occurs in association with other diseases (see below).

Ankylosing spondylitis has been thought of as a male disease, with the ratio of men to women approximately ten to one, but more recent research suggests that the sexes may be almost equally involved, with women generally having more mild cases. Some physicians are still unaware of this and are reluctant to make the diagnosis of ankylosing spondylitis in females. In many women the spine disease can be quite subtle, leading to a lengthy delay before the correct diagnosis is made.

Arthritis Associated with Inflammatory Bowel Disease

This may sound like a rather strange association, but approximately ten to twenty percent of patients with diseases that cause inflammation of the intestine, such as ulcerative colitis and regional enteritis, may suffer from a coexisting arthritis. The latter can take many forms, the most common of which involves the knee, ankle, elbow, wrist, or shoulder joints. This type of involvement waxes and wanes along with the activity of the bowel disease; that is, it flares when the bowel disease is active and remits when the bowel disease improves. It may last for weeks to months at a time.

Some patients with inflammatory bowel disease also suffer from ankylosing spondylitis. Unlike the arthritis described above, the spondylitis runs an independent course and may be active when the bowel disease is quiet and vice versa.

Arthritis Caused by Infections

A number of infectious agents are capable of causing arthritis. In the "old days," joints were commonly infected by tuberculosis; now they are infected by a number of bacterial organisms, one of the more common of which is gonorrhea.

Various viruses cause arthritis. Most common are the viruses responsible for hepatitis, mumps, and German measles, or rubella. The latter is especially interesting, because vaccines administered to prevent German measles have been known to cause arthritis. Although the arthritis is most often short-lived, usually lasting under one week and occasionally a few months, it has sometimes recurred and on rare occasions has lasted for a number of years. As the rubella vaccines have been refined, arthritis has become less of a problem. Permanent joint damage almost certainly does not occur in this condition. Women in their child-bearing years should be made immune from rubella infection since infection during pregnancy can lead to severe birth defects. A blood test determines if you are immune. Pregnancy should be delayed for three months after vaccination. You should discuss the advisability of this vaccination with your physician if you have any doubts or fears.

Even viruses responsible for common cases of the flu cause joint aches and pains, but this is a transient condition.

One of the most recently discovered forms of arthritis caused by an infection is called Lyme disease. Originally described in 1975, it is named after the town of Old Lyme, Connecticut, where the original cases occurred. It is caused by an organism called a spirochete, which is transmitted by the bites of deer ticks and mouse ticks. Lyme disease can be contracted in any tick-infested area but is most common in the Northeast from Massachusetts to Maryland, in the Midwest, especially in Wisconsin and Minnesota, and in the West, especially in California and Oregon. Lyme disease most commonly has its onset between May 1 and November 30, with peaks in June and July.

The illness usually begins with a rash, which expands around the area of the bite. Since the ticks are so small, many people do not recall being bitten. The rash is often accompanied by fatigue, fever, chills, and headache. These are flu-like symptoms; be wary when they occur in the summer or early fall, unusual times for flu to strike.

The arthritis develops within a few weeks to two years after the onset of Lyme disease and occurs in approximately sixty percent of patients. Other areas of the body, such as the heart and nervous system, may also be involved.

It is important that this disease be diagnosed, as it can usually be successfully treated with antibiotics. If you've been camping in the woods or been to an area where there is a deer population and develop any of the above symptoms, you may have Lyme disease. Since the arthritis may not appear until the other symptoms have disappeared, don't forget to tell your doctor about recent illnesses, even if you think they are trivial.

Lyme disease also occurs in pets and farm animals such as cows and horses. If you have an animal with joint problems, fever, and/or poor appetite, see your veterinarian. Lyme disease in animals may be the first clue that the illness is in your area.

Finally, in this day and age AIDS is obviously a major concern. Emerging research suggests that people with AIDS may develop various types of arthritis as the AIDS virus impairs the normal functioning of the immune system. The majority of these people develop the arthritis late in the disease, once the diagnosis is clear.

Gout

No disease has been as extensively written about as gout. References date from the 5th century B.C., when Hippocrates chronicled what would become known as the "disease of kings" because of its association with the "good life" — an excess of fine food and drink. This type of arthritis gained most of its notoriety in the England of Tom Jones with its wanton feasts.

Gout is associated with an abnormally high level of uric acid in the blood. This substance is a waste product derived from the breakdown of substances found in foods called purines. Examples of purine-rich foods include organ meats such as kidney and liver, anchovies, and sardines. Normally the uric acid is dissolved in the blood and eliminated from the body by the kidneys.

An elevated blood uric acid level, termed *hyperuricemia,* is caused by a decreased ability of the kidney to eliminate uric acid, increased production of uric acid by the body, or a combination of the two.

In people with gout, some of the uric acid precipitates into crystals, which are deposited in joints and other tissues. They may be deposited under the skin. Each deposit is called a *tophus.* Sometimes these crystals migrate and are shed into the joint space. The crystals irritate the joint lining and inflammation ensues.

It is sometimes necessary to remove fluid from an involved joint to make the diagnosis of gout. The fluid is examined under a microscope for the presence of uric acid crystals.

Episodes of gout can be triggered by excessive ingestion of food or alcohol, although most people with gout do not have to alter their diets significantly. Crash diets, trauma, joint injuries, surgery, and severe illnesses are other precipitating events. Often there is no obvious cause.

Attacks are self-limited; that is, even when untreated, they seldom last more than a few weeks. They are usually separated by months or even years. In some patients, the interval between attacks begins to shorten. Rarely, one acute attack ends where the next begins. The result is then chronic joint pain. Repeated attacks are usually necessary to damage joints. Some people experience "mini-attacks," which last for only a few hours to a few days and are deceptively mild. The area most often affected is the base of the large toe, the location where bunions occur. Other frequently involved joints include the feet, ankles, knees, and wrists, although almost any joint may be involved.

Hyperuricemia is not synonymous with gout; in fact, although it has been estimated that as many as five percent of Americans have elevated uric acid levels, less than twenty percent of those will ultimately develop gout. Some patients with gout have a normal uric acid level. An increased level of uric acid may be caused by diuretics, which are medications used to rid the body of excess fluid and to treat high blood pressure. Many diuretics decrease the kidneys' ability to remove uric acid, thus increasing the level in the blood.

Gout is predominantly a disease of males, with the peak age of onset approximately 50. It is extremely rare in premenopausal females. It occasionally runs in families. It may be associated with a number of other medical problems, including obesity, diabetes, and high blood pressure. Sometimes uric acid is deposited in the kidneys, causing kidney stones.

It is fortunate that gout is relatively easy to treat because it can cause the most severe arthritic pain. In 1683 Thomas Sydenham, a famous English physician often referred to as the English Hippocrates, vividly described an episode of gout:

> The victim goes to bed and sleeps in good health. About two o'clock in the morning he is awakened by a severe pain in the great toe; more rarely in the heel, ankle or instep. This pain is like that of a dislocation, and yet the parts feel as if cold water were poured over them. Then follow chills and shivers and a little fever. The pain, which was at first moderate, becomes more intense. With its intensity the chills and fever increase . . . Now it is a violent stretching and tearing of the ligaments — now it is a gnawing pain and now a pressure and tightening. So exquisite and lively meanwhile is the feeling of the part affected that it cannot bear the weight of bedclothes

nor the jar of a person walking in the room. The night is passed in torture, sleeplessness, turning of the part affected, and perpetual change of posture; the tossing about of the body being as incessant as the pain of the tortured joint . . .

It sounds unbearable, and it is — joint pain so bad that even the pressure of an overlying sheet is often intolerable. There is no reason to put up with this situation. Attacks of gout can be treated and, with certain medications, even prevented — another reason to see your doctor if you've been experiencing joint pain.

Fibromyalgia

This condition is also called fibrositis. It occurs most commonly in women of child-bearing age, and there is increasing evidence that it may begin in the teens. It is seen less often in males and postmenopausal females. It is being seen with increased frequency, and some rheumatologists claim it is one of the most common diseases they see.

Patients with fibromyalgia experience pain and aching in their muscles and joints, a general feeling of stiffness, and varying degrees of fatigue. Some people complain of numbness and tingling and of "poor circulation," although there is nothing objectively wrong with their circulation. Numerous discrete areas of tenderness called *trigger points* are located in various muscles and bones. Sometimes patients are unaware of their presence and express surprise when the physician locates them. Other than the presence of the trigger points, the results of the physical examination are normal. Even though joints may ache, they are not overtly warm, red, or swollen.

Fibromyalgia is often hard to diagnose. No laboratory tests can detect it, and unless the physician is familiar with it and knows where to look for the trigger points, the physical examination will also fail to reveal the condition. Under these circumstances the patient is often thought to be malingering or to have psychoneurotic problems. Indeed, this condition is often misdiagnosed, although less so of late as physicians become more aware of its existence. The diagnostic situation may be further complicated because fibromyalgia sometimes coexists with diseases such as rheumatoid arthritis.

Many patients with fibromyalgia have what is termed a *sleep disorder*. They may have difficulty falling asleep or sleep very lightly and awaken frequently during the course of the night. They awaken feeling tired and unrefreshed. The severity of the sleep disturbance appears to correlate with morning stiffness and fatigue.

Fibrositis pain appears to be worsened by overexertion, stress, and cold, damp weather. It is usually helped by a good exercise program and improvement in the sleep disorder.

The illness is unpredictable in its duration and can last many years. On a brighter note, our understanding of its treatment has improved considerably, and in my experience most people can be significantly helped.

A host of other conditions are associated with arthritis. These include blood abnormalities such as hemophilia and sickle cell anemia, various hormone abnormalities, and a group of diseases characterized by abnormalities of the immune system, often called autoimmune diseases. Rheumatoid arthritis is in the last category, as are such illnesses as systemic lupus erythematosus, or lupus for short, and scleroderma. A number of arthritic diseases occur in children as well.

There are countless other illnesses that afflict the joints. But the main purpose of this book is not to serve as a medical textbook, but rather to present a practical approach to arthritis, no matter what the cause. Thus it suffices to describe the more common types of arthritis as a background for the chapters that follow.

Before proceeding, however, there is one additional basic question that is commonly asked.

Can any joint develop arthritis?

The answer to this question is a qualified yes. Certainly any area customarily considered a joint can become arthritic. This includes virtually all the moveable and semimoveable joints. A number of examples follow.

Sacroiliac Joint

As noted above, the sacroiliac joints are located in the low back, over the area of the upper buttocks. They are involved in a number of inflammatory conditions such as ankylosing spondylitis, but osteoarthritis occasionally occurs in these joints as well.

The Spine

The spine is a rather complicated structure. It consists of twenty-four individual bones, called *vertebrae,* which are joined at *facet joints.* The vertebrae are separated from one another by an elastic material called a *disc,* which serves as a cushion or shock absorber.

The spinal cord is strung through the vertebrae, much as string is run through beads in a necklace. Nerves exit the spinal cord at the level of each vertebra and then extend to the various parts of the body. An elaborate network of muscles, tendons, and ligaments surrounds the spine, lending additional support.

Inflammation of the joints between the vertebral bodies can result in pain anywhere along the spine, from the neck down to the lower back. As noted above, inflammatory conditions such as ankylosing spondylitis and the spondylitis associated with inflammatory bowel disease and psoriasis may involve the spine. Like the sacroiliac joint, the spine is also subject to osteoarthritis.

However, there are many other causes of back pain. A disc may rupture, compressing the surrounding nerves and causing back pain and discomfort that radiates down one or both legs and sometimes into the foot. This may occur after trauma, bending, or lifting, or be unassociated with a specific precipitating event.

As we grow older the discs may degenerate. This is called *degenerative disc disease* and is often associated with back pain.

Older individuals with degenerative disc disease and osteoarthritis may develop a condition called *spinal stenosis,* in which a combination of factors results in narrowing of the canal through which the spinal cord passes. This causes pressure on the nerves, which may produce back pain as well as pain, weakness, or numbness in the legs. Typically the pain of spinal stenosis worsens with walking and is relieved by rest.

Spasm of the supporting muscles of the spine and sprained ligaments may also cause pain.

In addition, the individual vertebral bodies may collapse, or fracture, as a result of trauma. In the presence of osteoporosis, a thinning of the bones that occurs as we grow older, they may collapse spontaneously. This is often quite painful.

A number of factors, including excess weight, poor posture, lack of exercise, and stress, may contribute to back pain as well.

This is just a brief list of problems that can develop in the back. In addition, back pain may be caused by a number of medical conditions such as prostate problems in men, abnormalities of the uterus or ovaries in women, kidney problems, and abnormalities in the digestive system.

Thus back and neck pain may be due to

a number of conditions, including arthritis. See your doctor if the pain is severe, has been present for more than six weeks despite home remedies, or is accompanied by weakness, numbness, or pain in one or both legs; if there is a change in bladder or bowel habits; if the pain resulted from trauma; or if it is accompanied by other problems such as fever, abdominal pain, or loss of appetite.

Costochondral Joint

These joints are located where the ribs join the breastbone, or sternum. Inflammation of these joints is termed costochondritis and occurs in ankylosing spondylitis and in the arthritis associated with inflammatory bowel disease and psoriasis and can cause severe chest pain. Sometimes the arthritis is unassociated with other conditions.

Temporomandibular Joint

This is simply a fancy term for the jaw, another area not traditionally thought of as a joint. Yet it is, and it can be involved in various types of arthritis, such as rheumatoid arthritis. Poor alignment of teeth or a poorly fitting bridge can cause temporomandibular arthritis.

Temporomandibular joint syndrome, or TMJ syndrome, is the term used when the jaw doesn't function properly. Individuals with TMJ syndrome often have a number of complaints — tenderness over the jaw, a grating or clicking sound when opening or closing the mouth, locking of the jaw, and jaw pain when chewing or yawning. TMJ syndrome may also be associated with a number of other, less obvious complaints such as a headache, earache, and dizziness.

Any problem associated with the temporomandibular joint, with the ligaments around the jaw, or with the muscles responsible for chewing can cause TMJ syndrome. Most of the symptoms are probably caused by spasm of the chewing muscles. In addition to arthritis and local misalignment within the mouth, TMJ syndrome is also caused by accidents to the jaw, head, or neck and by clenching or grinding the teeth.

Cricoarytenoid Joints

These small joints are located in the throat and move with the vocal cords to vary the pitch and tone of the voice. They occasionally become arthritic, especially in the patient with rheumatoid arthritis. In fact, it has been estimated that almost one third of patients with rheumatoid arthritis have involvement of these joints. When the problem is severe enough, hoarseness may result.

If you have rheumatoid or some other form of arthritis and have noticed hoarseness, inform your doctor. If the problem doesn't act like typical laryngitis and clear up within a relatively short period of time, you may very well have "arthritis of the throat." This is often treated successfully, usually by local sprays.

Why do people get arthritis in the first place? This is discussed in the next chapter.

4

The Search for Answers

Knowledge is power.
— FRANCIS BACON

We all have a basic need to control our destinies; an understanding of why things went wrong helps us accomplish this. Unfortunately, because of our need to know, conclusions that have not been scientifically validated are often offered to a public that wants easy answers to complex problems.

In this chapter we'll discuss theories regarding the causes of arthritis and explode a few myths in the process.

The first question, stark in its simplicity and directness, is one of those most commonly asked of any physician.

Why did this happen to me?

Usually the answer to this question is an honest "I don't know." Certainly there are some arthritic diseases, such as Lyme arthritis, with an obvious cause, but they are in the minority. More often than not, modern medicine simply cannot explain why one person develops arthritis and another does not. However, we often have at least partial explanations.

For example, many forms of arthritis appear to be hereditary; that is, they run in families. Ankylosing spondylitis, rheumatoid arthritis, gout, and osteoarthritis (see Chapter 3 for additional causes of osteoarthritis) all seem to fit into this category to varying degrees. Yet it is impossible to predict which family members will develop a specific disease.

In some cases, specific genes have been recognized as being more common in patients with particular illnesses. The best example of this is ankylosing spondylitis. Approximately ninety percent of people who suffer from this disease possess a gene termed HLA B 27. About eight percent of the white population and four percent of the black population possess this gene. The presence of the gene is obviously important, but it isn't the entire explanation. Studies of identical twins possessing the HLA B 27 gene indicate that if one twin develops spondylitis the other twin may not. Similarly, no more than twenty percent of people with the HLA B 27 gene develop the disease. Finally, HLA B 27–positive relatives of HLA B 27–positive individuals with ankylosing spondylitis are more likely to develop ankylosing spondylitis than are HLA B 27–positive relatives of HLA B 27–positive individuals who are healthy.

Similar but less compelling information is available regarding rheumatoid arthritis. Rheumatoid arthritis appears to run in families, and identical twins are both more likely to develop the disease than are nonidentical twins. As with ankylosing spondylitis, a specific gene — in this case the DR4 gene — appears to be associated with rheumatoid arthritis. The risk of developing rheumatoid arthritis is greater in individuals who possess the gene than in those who do not, but only a minority are affected.

The arthritis that is associated with psoriasis is also associated with specific genes (it has been known for years that psoriasis runs in families). Although some cases of osteo-arthritis, especially those involving the hands and feet, appear to run in families, a specific gene association has yet to be identified. Gout is also considered a hereditary disease, but again, a specific gene has not been identified.

It is clear that an individual's genetic makeup alone is not responsible for the development of arthritis. What, then, is the cause? Most researchers currently theorize that arthritis develops when the body's immune system does not respond normally when exposed to something foreign, such as bacteria or a virus. This triggers an immune response, which means that inflammation occurs in various parts of the body, including the joints. In other words, a large group of people could all be exposed to the same bacteria; some of those who possess a certain gene, which tells the immune system how to react, would ultimately develop arthritis; for the most part, the others would not. This has been demonstrated in the case of people with the HLA B 27 gene. When they are exposed to specific bacterial agents — for example, salmonella or shigella, both of which cause diarrhea — approximately twenty percent go on to develop an arthritic disease similar to ankylosing spondylitis called Reiter's syndrome.

Under normal circumstances, the immune system protects the body against invasion from outside factors, such as bacteria and viruses. When foreign organisms invade the body, they are packaged by various elements of the immune system to form *antigens*. The immune system then makes *antibodies* to fight the antigens. Sometimes the body is tricked into thinking that part of itself is actually foreign and manufacturing antibodies directed against itself. These are called *autoantibodies,* and the illnesses in which these occur are called *autoimmune diseases.* Many rheumatic diseases, including rheumatoid arthritis and systemic lupus erythematosus, are classified as auto-immune diseases.

Finally, one patient's rheumatoid arthritis may have a hereditary basis, while the next person's may not. It may take many generations for a particular juxtaposition of circumstances to occur and result in arthritis. Therefore, if your parents and grandparents did not have the disease, it does not necessarily mean you are protected. In addition, arthritis in a given person may not have a hereditary basis at all — thus family history may be of little importance.

Besides being concerned about where they got their arthritis, many people are equally concerned about their children's chances of developing the disease. Although there are statistics suggesting that possession of the genes previously discussed indicates an increased chance of developing arthritis, this is by no means a certainty, or even a likelihood. Even if you, your parents, and your grandparents have a certain type of arthritis, it still doesn't mean your children will get it.

Could I have done anything to prevent it?

The answers to the preceding questions have

shown that most people cannot prevent the development of their arthritis. It is important that people with arthritis realize they aren't at fault and channel their energies into getting better, not into remorse and self-blame. As we shall see, our emotional state is a key factor in determining whether we get the better of our disease or it gets the better of us. We want to make our emotions an ally, not an enemy.

This vital point reminds me of Richard Gorton, a 39-year-old man who had always been healthy until being struck with rheumatoid arthritis. A successful businessman, he had decided to celebrate his most recent triumphs by taking his entire family on vacation. So, accompanied by his wife, two children, his parents, his in-laws, and an aunt and uncle, he left for two weeks in Paris.

Within three days of their arrival the entire family was ill, devastated by severe nausea, vomiting, diarrhea, aches, and fever. On average, the illness lasted between 36 and 48 hours. All recovered — except Richard. Although his gastrointestinal symptoms disappeared, he continued to ache.

On his return from this aborted trip Richard saw his internist, who, alarmed by the continuing symptoms, suggested he see a rheumatologist and referred him to me. By the time

I saw him, Richard was experiencing joint pain that was beginning to interfere with his everyday life. He was so stiff in the morning that routine tasks took an inordinate amount of time. He was often late for work and too tired to keep his usual long hours. He'd previously exercised three times a week but now couldn't at all. He was so uncomfortable at night he had difficulty sleeping.

When I asked Richard what was wrong, he said, "I feel like I got the flu and it never went away." This is a common feeling when patients first develop rheumatoid arthritis — which is exactly what he had. When I told him what his problem was, he looked at me blankly. I proceeded to explain my treatment plan, trying to be as encouraging and upbeat as possible, but it was clear he didn't really hear what I was saying.

I prescribed an anti-inflammatory medication and physical therapy and asked him to return in one month. At that time he was no better, which surprised and alarmed me since most people improve noticeably once treatment is begun. I changed his medication and asked him to call me in two weeks. When he did, he was still no better. Again I tried to be encouraging and increased his medication.

I only had to look into his face to realize

he had not improved by his next visit. We were both getting frustrated. My first words to him were quite general. "Richard, what's wrong?"

He answered promptly, seemingly without thinking. "I should never have gone on that trip," he said. "This never would have happened if I just stayed home." He didn't talk about his joints, about how he felt, only about his vacation. He fixated on it — he couldn't get it out of his mind. A man who was successful in everything he did, who controlled his own destiny better than most of us, he couldn't come to grips with the reality of his disease.

When Richard remarked on how the trip had ruined his life, I told him it would only do so if he allowed it to. I further explained that he could have developed rheumatoid arthritis elsewhere, under other circumstances. I don't know if he would have, but I can't say he wouldn't have either. At any rate he was so caught up with what he couldn't change that it dominated what he could change. He needed emotional as well as physical help. An insightful person, he soon recognized his need for counseling. After a few sessions, his fixation with the trip diminished, and he finally began to improve physically as well.

Richard Gorton still has rheumatoid arthritis. Thanks to modern medicine, he is in almost complete remission and has returned to his prior lifestyle. But his success is only partially attributable to modern medicine. Richard's frame of mind is as responsible for his well-being as any drug I've ever given him.

Does stress cause arthritis?

The more we learn about the interrelationship between stress and the immune system, the more complicated this question becomes. In the "old days" of medicine, most practitioners drew a line separating the mind and the body. Lately that line has become hazy, and in many people's minds it has disappeared.

Stress clearly worsens organic or "physical" problems. For example, heart disease occurs when fat accumulations narrow the walls of the arteries that deliver oxygen to the heart, thus reducing blood flow. Increased physical activity puts extra demands on the heart, increasing its need for oxygen. If those needs can't be met, the heart does not receive enough oxygen, and pain, or angina, results. Yet angina also occurs in response to stress.

Numerous other examples could be given to illustrate the relationship between emotional well-being and organic diseases. For example, patients with broken limbs admitted to hospitals heal more rapidly and are discharged more quickly when the professional staff makes an active effort to improve their emotional well-being.

It therefore comes as no great surprise that *stress worsens arthritis.* In some way we don't completely understand, it affects the immune and hormonal systems, which in turn affect the joint disease. It probably has an adverse effect on all types of arthritis, including osteoarthritis and rheumatoid arthritis. Stress probably plays a role in the development and perception of pain as well.

Although many investigators are in agreement that stress worsens arthritis, few are willing to say that stress causes it. If large groups of patients with rheumatoid arthritis are studied, it is apparent that a stressful event preceded development of the arthritis in a significant number of them. On the other hand, stress is such a common part of all of our lives that it is unclear whether this relationship is coincidental or more significant.

The relationship between stress and arthritis is dramatically illustrated by the case of actress Jane Withers. At the age of 27, between her motion picture career and her first commercials as Josephine, the lady plumber, her marriage began to unravel. Burdened by marital pressures as well as the responsibilities of caring for her children, she developed severe rheumatoid arthritis. She was in the hospital for months, unable to walk and at times even unable to turn over in bed without help.

Refusing to believe she would be permanently incapacitated, she supplemented her medical care with positive thoughts, which included imagining herself walking and dancing again. And she did do those things.

Unfortunately, more bouts of arthritis followed. Jane remarried, and this time things went well. She and her husband built a new house. The day before they were to move in, he was killed in a plane crash. Within 48 hours her arthritis was back. She has vivid memories of her knuckles starting to get red and swollen and yelling at them, "No way are you going to do this to me again." She survived that bout in much the same manner as she survived the first — with good medical care and by using a number of methods to reduce the enormous stress in her life. When stressed, her joints still "act up," but she is in control. Her strategy of reducing stress and obtaining proper medical treatment has stood her in good stead.

Now Jane Withers is a spokesperson for a senior citizens' self-help group. She urges her audiences to stimulate their minds while taking care of their bodies. Her motto, "You can do anything," seems particularly apropos after hearing her story.

Dancer Donna McKechnie's story is somewhat similar. In 1975 she was the star of the hit Broadway musical *A Chorus Line*. In 1977 she married choreographer Michael Bennett. The marriage was a stormy one and soon ended in divorce. Her joints began to ache as the marriage went downhill. In her own words, "They blew up after the divorce was finalized." The diagnosis was rheumatoid arthritis.

She went from playing Cassie, the main character in *A Chorus Line,* to virtual immobility. "My rheumatoid arthritis came on after a list of losses. My father died, I got a divorce, and I lost a job." To add insult to injury, her doctors told her she would never dance again. Donna McKechnie was soon in a deep depression.

She went into intensive psychotherapy and used yoga to reduce stress. Her joints slowly improved, and she began to exercise. They got even better, and she started to dance again. Just a little at first, then some more. She went back to work, initially appearing in parts that were not physically challenging. Her confidence buoyed by her success, her joints even better, in 1989 she once again starred as

Cassie, in a three-month road tour of *A Chorus Line*. Her joints still ache on occasion, especially when she is tired. But at the age of 46, she says, "I'm stronger now than when I was thirty."

Did stress cause Jane Withers' or Donna McKechnie's arthritis? I spoke with Dr. Malcolm Rogers, assistant professor of psychiatry at Harvard Medical School, who is an authority on stress. "A number of studies have been done which link stress to the immune system," he says. However, he adds, there is not enough hard scientific information at present to justify the conclusion that there is an irrefutable cause-and-effect relationship between stress and the development of arthritis. For now, most health care professionals agree that stress aggravates arthritis and occasionally unmasks it in a susceptible individual.

Did positive thoughts help Jane Withers get better? What role did Donna McKechnie's psychotherapy and yoga play? Dr. Rogers says, "The greater the extent to which people think they influence the course of their disease, the better off they are." The more helpless people feel, the worse they do. The more they get involved and do things to help themselves, the better they do. Jane Withers helped herself. So did Donna McKechnie. A positive attitude is an essential ingredient to recovery.

In our continuing quest to discover why people develop arthritis, the role of diet is often questioned. This question takes many forms.

Is arthritis caused by something in my diet? Is it caused by a dietary deficiency, such as a vitamin deficiency? Is it caused by a food allergy?

There is a lot of confusion regarding the relationship between diet and arthritis. Is this another example of believing what we want to believe, especially if that belief somehow empowers us to control our fate? Or is there validity to the opinion that diet influences arthritis?

There is certainly a considerable precedent regarding the relationship between diet and disease. It is difficult to pick up a magazine or newspaper without reading about the link between cholesterol and heart disease. Similarly, relationships between diet and various types of cancer clearly exist. In addition, it seems logical that diet influences all aspects of our well-being — after all, "We are what we eat."

On theoretical grounds, diet may influence arthritis in a number of ways. Diet may predispose the patient to develop arthritis, much as a high-fat diet is a risk factor for the development of cancer of the colon. Diet may also have a direct effect on the immune system, either by allowing arthritis to develop or by compromising the body's ability to fight it. Finally, some people may be allergic to certain foods, and this allergy may produce an attack of arthritis or worsen a pre-existing arthritic condition.

Indeed, various studies have demonstrated that some patients with rheumatoid arthritis improve while fasting or on low-fat, low-protein, low-calorie diets. The improvement is usually minor, and we're not sure why it occurs.

Other studies suggest that changes in diet may help arthritis. However, they are preliminary and involve relatively small groups of people. Much more needs to be done before irrefutable conclusions can be drawn.

Donna McKechnie is convinced that changing her diet was one of the factors that improved her arthritis. Is she correct? I don't know, but I think we should all be as open-minded as possible — on both sides of the issue. Even Donna says, "I think it helped me, but that doesn't mean it will help everyone."

Interestingly, many patients are convinced that various foods aggravate their arthritis. However, when these people are tested in a scientific fashion, their observations rarely hold up. A few people do indeed correctly identify a culpable food substance in their diet, usually milk or another dairy product. When the offending food is eliminated, the arthritis improves or disappears. When it is returned, the arthritis flares. However, as stated, this represents a minority of patients.

I will never forget a woman in her mid-50s who consulted me because of an unusual medical condition called palindromic rheumatism. This is what doctors call an episodic, self-limited form of arthritis, which means that it comes and goes at various intervals, usually days to weeks at a time. It is often quite severe, can be temporarily debilitating, and is quite unpredictable. Because it appears and disappears quickly, there is a tendency to look for causes, to relate the development of the arthritis to specific events in the patient's life.

When I initially interviewed this patient, one of the first things she said was that she was allergic to tomatoes. When asked to explain, she said she rarely ate fresh tomatoes, but did so the night before her first attack. When she awakened the following morning with a number of swollen joints, she automatically assumed she was having an allergic reaction, and the most likely culprit was tomatoes.

By the time I saw her, the attack was over and she was feeling quite well. However, she wanted to know what allergy medicine to take should she experience another episode. I explained that it was unlikely a food allergy was responsible for her arthritis, and suggested an anti-inflammatory drug should there be a recurrence. She was skeptical, but agreed to see me again.

Upon her return a month later, she said she had experienced another episode of arthritis, this one beginning the morning after eating a Swiss cheese sandwich — an unusual meal for her. Now she was allergic to Swiss cheese, and wouldn't even consider an alternate explanation. In fact, if I wouldn't prescribe an allergy medicine she wouldn't come back to see me. I didn't, and she said she'd let me know if she needed me.

A number of months passed. Finally, quite by accident, I met her on the street in front of the hospital where I work. I asked how she was feeling. "Doctor," she answered, "you'll be surprised to hear I'm allergic to more foods than I originally thought." She then proceeded to name virtually every food she had eaten before an attack of arthritis —

everything from watermelon to blueberry pie. It took an additional year and countless attacks before she became convinced she had arthritis, not food allergies. Thankfully, she is currently receiving appropriate therapy and doing quite well. She's even eating blueberry pie.

In summary, there is no global evidence to suggest that a specific food product, including vitamins, causes or cures arthritis. The only possible exception to this is fish oils, which may help rheumatoid arthritis (more on this in Chapter 11).

I've seen a number of patients who were convinced their diet influenced their arthritis, but only one bore up under scrutiny. Margo Enninger was a 33-year-old woman with rheumatoid arthritis who was absolutely certain her disease was worsened by dairy products such as milk and ice cream. In fact, she was so steadfast in her belief that she consulted me as a third, not second, opinion. The first two rheumatologists she saw were so skeptical of her observation that she thought they belittled her. Since an ideal doctor–patient relationship involves a healthy amount of give and take, she felt she couldn't continue under those doctors' care.

When I saw her, I also expressed doubt about her observation but was quick to add that patients respond in a number of individual and unique fashions, and we should try to be as unprejudiced as possible. Note that I said "we" should be unprejudiced, as she had to consider the possibility she was wrong too.

We agreed she would eliminate dairy products from her diet. I examined her when she thought she was doing relatively well, making special note of the degree of swelling and tenderness in her joints. She then began to drink milk regularly and returned in two weeks. At that time she complained of increased pain and stiffness, and on physical examination I found that her joints were significantly more tender and swollen than they had been previously.

Did she improve because she thought she would, or did the milk and ice cream truly affect her arthritis? Or was it something else altogether? I've known this woman for a number of years, and it does indeed appear as if her arthritis is directly influenced by dairy products. Yet as stated, she is clearly the exception.

Is it folly to think that at least some improvement after dietary manipulation is due to a placebo effect? Consider the following.

Early in my career I was privileged to be exposed to some of the giants of American rheumatology, people who helped establish rheumatology as a subspecialty and did a significant amount of the pioneering research.

One dreary Friday afternoon I had a snack with one of them in the hospital cafeteria. Both of our clinic patients had cancelled their appointments, and serendipity brought us together over a cup of coffee.

Always eager to pick the brains of the old professors, I asked him how he approached patients with rheumatoid arthritis who were not doing as well as expected. Bear in mind that our options were much more limited in those days. I was simply expecting to hear his views on dose schedules of medications and combining various commonly used drugs. His answer surprised me.

"I'll tell you something I never would have told you while you were in training," he said and smiled — a reference to his belief that trainees should learn "by the book" but that knowledge of the real art of medicine would follow much later. I sat expectantly, eager for his pearls of wisdom.

"Vitamins," he said. "When they don't do well, I give them vitamins. And when that doesn't work I start fooling around with their diet. Usually ask them to stop eating something, maybe red meat, especially if they're eating too much of that anyway." (This conversation preceded our knowledge of cholesterol by years.)

"But none of those things are supposed to work," I blurted out, somewhat flabbergasted.

"I know," he responded, "but they can't hurt. And if you really can convince the patient they'll work, you know something? They will. Besides, what else do you have to offer them?"

With that he downed his last mouthful of coffee, got up from the table, and walked back to the clinic. And we never discussed it again — it was almost as if the conversation never happened.

Did this renowned physician know something the rest of us didn't? Perhaps he did, but I don't know if it had anything to do with diet and arthritis. It did have to do with motivation, and wanting to get better, and we could all use a little more of that.

In summary, there is presently insufficient evidence to warrant a specific diet to treat your arthritis. However, it is important that you follow sound dietary principles, as discussed in Chapter 10.

Finally, a question some people regard as comical, others an old wives' tale.

Does cracking your knuckles lead to arthritis?

For years most rheumatologists dismissed this

as myth. A recent study, however, revealed that knuckle-cracking may be associated with hand weakness and swelling. Even though this has not yet been verified by additional studies, cracking your knuckles may be a good habit to break!

With this bit of perspective, it is apparent that anything from your genetic makeup to a nervous habit may be related to the development of arthritis. This demonstrates the need for further research so that arthritis will eventually join diseases such as polio and smallpox in near extinction.

Now we will travel from the theoretical to the concrete — the symptoms of arthritis.

5

The Symptoms of Arthritis

The symptoms of arthritis can be quite complex and confusing, but we'll start with the basics.

What are the symptoms of arthritis?

Since arthritis is a joint disease, most of the symptoms involve the joints. The main symptoms are pain and stiffness. The pain is described in different ways. Some patients say their joints ache, others say they burn. Others say they feel as if they have a sprain; still others say the pain is so bad it feels like a broken bone.

Stiffness is usually most prominent in the morning and is a helpful symptom to the physician. It is referred to as *morning stiffness,* and it helps differentiate the two major classes of arthritis, osteoarthritis, or degenerative joint disease, and inflammatory types of arthritis, such as rheumatoid arthritis. Patients with the former normally experience relatively brief amounts of morning stiffness, usually less than half an hour. Patients with inflammatory arthritis are usually stiff for at least thirty to forty-five minutes or more. There is obviously a gray zone, and it is not always possible to delineate the two categories of arthritis on the basis of this symptom. The degree of morning stiffness also helps the physician determine the severity of the inflammation. For example, a patient with two hours of morning stiffness is more severely afflicted than an individual with one hour of stiffness. Similarly, morning stiffness can be used as a barometer to help determine the efficacy of therapy. If before treatment a patient complained of three hours of stiffness, and one medication reduced it to two hours while another reduced it to one hour, the second drug is obviously more effective.

Some patients do not use the word *stiffness* when describing their morning discomfort. They may say their joints feel fatigued, painful, swollen, or simply don't feel right. Individuals with osteoarthritis go on to say that once their morning stiffness disappears, they usually feel well *until they become active.* Although an appropriate amount of activity, usually in the form of exercise, often results in a lessening of discomfort, excessive activity, the definition of which varies from patient to patient, usually causes increased pain, either during the activity or after it ceases. This is also a good indicator of the severity of the arthritis. Joints that become painful after 2 hours of activity are more severely involved than joints that require three hours of activity to become painful. Sometimes the only evidence of overuse is increased stiffness or pain the following morning; that is, you may have to wait until Tuesday to find out if you did too much on Monday. This is an important principle, as it helps determine appropriate exercise levels. It will be discussed further in Chapters 9 and 10.

Patients with osteoarthritis usually say that rest eases the pain caused by arthritis. Again, the amount of rest required to reduce or eliminate pain is helpful in assessing the severity of the arthritis. Most patients improve markedly within a few hours. In some patients, osteoarthritic pain may be so severe that it extends into the night, making sleeping difficult. This is almost exclusively encountered in severely afflicted individuals.

Unlike patients with degenerative joint disease, once their morning stiffness abates, patients with inflammatory arthritis usually feel well *as long as they stay active.* They may still experience intermittent pain throughout the course of the day, but increased activity results in diminished discomfort as long as the patient doesn't do too much — then the pain will increase, just as it would in the patient with degenerative joint disease. Unfortunately, arthritis pain may also be quite unpredictable and almost seems to come and go as it pleases.

The relationship between activity and pain in osteoarthritis and rheumatoid arthritis also differs in degree. For example, patients with osteoarthritis of a knee generally feel better if they do some simple stretching exercises and take brief walks on a regular basis. However, lengthier walks predictably result in knee pain. On the other hand, patients with rheumatoid arthritis must remain significantly active in order to stay comfortable, although they can do too much as well.

Patients with inflammatory arthritis are in double jeopardy when they come down with simple problems such as the flu. The bed rest that this requires often results in worsening the symptoms of their arthritis. Patients with degenerative joint disease are not as severely afflicted.

Many patients with inflammatory arthritis, especially rheumatoid arthritis, say their stiffness returns later in the day despite their attempts to remain active. I will never forget the description of the daily pain and stiffness cycle given by a patient of mine with severe rheumatoid arthritis. She said she was extremely stiff upon arising, and this lasted until 2:00 in the afternoon. She felt relatively well from 2:00 to 3:00 P.M., and then her "evening" stiffness began. This lasted until she went to sleep. In other words, she only had one hour of relative comfort. This sad story has a happy ending, though. With a combination of drugs and physical therapy (which will be discussed in Chapters 8 and 9), she has done well and now only experiences an hour of stiffness in the morning and none in the afternoon!

Patients with both types of arthritis may experience stiffness after episodes of inactivity. Sitting in an automobile for a prolonged period of time or sitting through a movie or long dinner may result in increased stiffness. My patients sometimes tell me I'm responsible for their stiffness if I make them wait in my office for more than a few minutes, so I try to be on time!

In addition to pain and stiffness, individuals with arthritis may notice evidence of joint inflammation, such as swelling, redness, or warmth. Joints may be tender to the touch, and they may not move normally even though they may look normal.

The answer to the next question serves as a practical guide.

How do I know when my symptoms are severe enough to go to the doctor?

We all experience aches and pains on occasion. When do they warrant medical attention? If there is an obvious explanation for them, there is seldom cause for concern. For example, if you have exercised infrequently in the past and then begin an exercise program, it won't be surprising if you are uncomfortable. If you're a weekend athlete, getting no exercise during the week but playing anything from tennis to touch football on rare weekends, don't be surprised if you're uncomfortable that night or the next morning.

These aches and pains are *normal*. They shouldn't last too long, more than a day or so, or be very severe. Use your prior experiences as a source of reference. If the discomfort lasts longer or is more severe than usual, make an appointment to see your doctor.

Similarly, if you have discomfort that occurs in a reproducible fashion, see your physician. In other words, if you ache every time, or almost every time, you engage in a specific activity, especially one you're used to doing, you may be developing arthritis. If your joints are stiff in the morning, they may be inflamed. The stiffness may occur daily or periodically, perhaps three or four mornings a week. It may be precipitated by activities of the previous day that you don't perform on a routine basis, such as exercise or extra housework, then last for a number of mornings before disappearing, only to return under the same circumstances.

Athletes are very sensitive to changes in their bodies. Lynn Adams thinks her athletic experiences allowed her to differentiate early arthritic pain from the discomfort associated with exercise and activities. As she puts it, she has learned to separate "the good pain from the bad pain" and emphasizes that the differences may be very subtle.

Francis Kelley, a rather astute 78-year-old man, consulted me because he noted right knee pain after walking for three miles. Mr. Kelley was as fit as men twenty to thirty years younger. He attributed his good health to his daily three-mile walk, which he had taken for years; it was only recently that his knee had begun to ache toward the end of the walk. On the rare days when he didn't walk, he had no discomfort. If he walked two and a half miles, he had no discomfort. But if he walked his usual three miles, he did. This was sufficiently unusual to motivate him to seek medical attention. He was diagnosed as having osteoarthritis, was successfully treated, and returned to his normal walking routine.

Mr. Kelley's discomfort was unusual *for*

him. Although many 78-year-old men will experience knee pain after walking three miles if they're not used to doing so, Mr. Kelley routinely engaged in this activity without difficulty. If the pain had only occurred a few times, he would not have sought medical attention. It was the combination of a new pain and its occurrence in a regular fashion that drove him to seek help.

In addition, the Arthritis Foundation has developed a list of warning signs of arthritis, which follows.

- Swelling in one or more joints
- Early morning stiffness
- Recurring pain or tenderness in any joint
- Inability to move a joint normally
- Obvious redness and warmth in a joint
- Unexplained weight loss, fever, or weakness combined with joint pain
- Symptoms such as these that last for more than two weeks.

If you have joint pains, consider the above before dismissing them as inconsequential. If your symptoms are severe, call your doctor as soon as possible. Even if you regard the discomfort as mild, see your doctor if it lasts for more than two weeks. The earlier you get help the better. And remember, as always, if you have any doubts, err on the side of caution and see your physician.

Once arthritic symptoms occur, will they always be the same?

The course of arthritis is often quite variable. At times you may feel relatively well, at others, poorly. This variability is most often seen in rheumatoid arthritis. Even patients with severe disease may have periods of time when they feel surprisingly well.

If the symptoms disappear, the disease is said to be in *remission*. If the disease returns or worsens, it is called a *flare*. Some patients with rheumatoid arthritis go into indefinite remission. This usually occurs within the first few years after onset of the disease.

It is important to realize that arthritic diseases do change. There may not necessarily be a cause-and-effect relationship between something you do or take and improvement in the arthritis. It may be a coincidence.

Now that we know about the symptoms of arthritis, what about related aches and pains? A typical question follows.

I have an ache in my upper arm, and my doctor told me it was from the arthritis in

my shoulder. How can that be?

This is called *referred pain,* the mechanism of which is poorly understood. In other words, even though the problem is in the shoulder, pain is perceived in the upper arm. Concurrent pain may or may not be present in the shoulder as well. Similarly, arthritis in the hip may be manifested by groin pain or discomfort in the upper leg. On occasion, hip pain is referred to the knee, even when the hip is entirely symptom-free. This is most often encountered in children and adolescents. Facial or ear pain may result from arthritis of the temporomandibular joint, or jaw. Headaches, especially those that occur in the back of the head, may come from arthritis of the neck.

In other words, the human body and its ailments can be exceedingly complicated. If you have a problem, go to your doctor — don't self-diagnose. The situation may be more complex than you think.

I have rheumatoid arthritis and have numbness in my hands, especially at night. Is that from the arthritis?

It is, but only indirectly. One of the nerves that goes to the hand is called the median nerve. It travels through a very narrow canal in the wrist called the carpal tunnel. Anything that results in swelling around the tunnel, such as the swelling from arthritis, causes increased pressure on the nerve. This may result in pain, numbness, and tingling in the involved hand. The symptoms are usually present in the thumb, index, middle, and part of the ring finger, but the entire hand may be involved. Pain may radiate back up the arm, sometimes all the way to the shoulder. Symptoms are worse at night and often awaken people from sleep. This is because most of us flex, or bend, our wrists when we sleep. This puts pressure on the carpal tunnel and the median nerve, and symptoms result. When people are awakened they usually shake or rub their hands to relieve the discomfort.

The most common causes of carpal tunnel syndrome are rheumatoid arthritis, the swelling that may result from pregnancy or birth control pills, and thyroid diseases. Activities that force the wrist to be bent for prolonged periods of time can result in carpal tunnel syndrome or worsen a preexisting problem. Simple activities such as holding a telephone, driving, typing, and writing may result in sufficient pressure on the nerve to cause symptoms.

The condition is treated in a number of ways, including splinting the wrist in order to decrease pressure on the nerve, injecting cortisone into the wrist to decrease swelling, and surgery.

The next few questions deal with various misconceptions concerning the symptoms of arthritis.

My joints ache but they look normal. Could I still have arthritis?

Definitely. Although joint inflammation is associated with redness, heat, pain, and swelling, the overt manifestations may be so subtle that you may not notice them. Occasionally your physician may be able to detect subtle evidence of inflammation through physical examination. In addition, various tests may detect inflammation that is not even evident on physical examination.

Conversely, the patient may, on occasion, be aware of an abnormality the physician can't detect. For example, many patients complain that their hands are swollen although they may look normal to their doctors.

Physicians who do not have significant experience with arthritis may discount their patients' complaints if they can't be substantiated on exam. Remember, it's your body; if it doesn't feel right to you, it probably isn't.

When my arthritis is active I feel more tired. Is that my imagination?

As discussed in Chapter 3, illnesses such as rheumatoid arthritis can affect the entire body. Fatigue is a major symptom of these diseases. Fatigue can in fact occur in patients with all types of arthritis. Pain wears people out, and they become physically and psychologically frustrated, which drains their energy. Frustration also occurs from the development of physical limitations. Painful joints can make sleeping difficult. This leads to increased fatigue as well. Depression may also play a role. The thought of having arthritis is depressing. Fears regarding loss of independence and body image may lead to depression. Depression in turn causes fatigue.

It is apparent that arthritis is not simply a joint disease, but rather an illness that can have pervasive effects on both mind and body.

Speaking of pervasive effects on the body leads us to the next question, an unusual one.

I went to my eye doctor because my eyes were dry and he told me I have arthritis of the eyes. What does that mean?

Arthritis of the eyes does not exist. We already know arthritis means inflammation of a joint, and the eye is obviously not a joint. However, dryness of the eyes, along with dryness of the mouth, may accompany diseases that involve the joints, such as rheumatoid arthritis and systemic lupus erythematosus. This condition of the eyes and mouth is called *Sjogren's syndrome,* and it can also occur by itself, without the presence of other illnesses. People with this problem complain of a number of symptoms, including dryness or burning of the eyes, blurry vision, and sometimes severe discomfort and pain. Another common complaint is the presence of excessive sandlike particles in the eyes upon arising in the morning. Still others feel as if they have foreign bodies in their eyes. Dryness of the mouth may result in difficulty chewing, swallowing, and speaking.

Dryness of the eyes is caused by inflammation of the lacrimal glands, which produce tears. Dryness of the mouth is caused by inflammation of the salivary glands. The inflammation prevents these glands from functioning normally, and the production of tears and saliva decreases. Decreased tear production sometimes results in damage to the cornea, which can be very painful. Similarly, decreased production of saliva can lead to the development of cavities, as normal amounts of saliva are necessary to protect teeth against decay. Thus the ophthalmologist (eye doctor) and dentist are important members of the team that cares for patients with illnesses such as rheumatoid arthritis.

The diagnosis of Sjogren's syndrome is made in a variety of ways. One is to measure tear production with a piece of filter paper. This is called the *Schirmer test*. Another is by doing a biopsy of the lip.

Eye discomfort is often relieved by the use of artificial tears. Dryness of the mouth necessitates frequent intake of fluids. Meticulous dental hygiene is important, and the use of sugar-free products is recommended.

Inflammation of other parts of the eye may also be found in association with rheumatoid arthritis, ankylosing spondylitis, lupus, and various types of arthritis in children. This may result in mild irritation of the lining of the eyes, scarring, glaucoma, and even decreased vision. Be sure to tell your eye doctor about your arthritis — it may prove helpful in making the correct diagnosis.

Now that we know about Sjogren's syndrome, the answer to the next question will make a bit more sense. It was asked by a 25-year-old woman with rheumatoid arthritis.

Ever since I developed rheumatoid arthritis I've had problems with vaginal burning and

dryness, which make sexual intercourse uncomfortable. Is this related to my arthritis?

These complaints are most probably also associated with Sjogren's syndrome. In addition to the lacrimal and salivary glands, the glands that supply moisture and lubrication to the skin of the external genitalia and vagina can also be involved in Sjogren's syndrome. This can lead to a burning sensation as well as *dyspareunia,* which is the medical term for painful intercourse. These symptoms are often alleviated by the application of various vaginal creams and jellies.

The following question addresses another unusual problem found in some patients with arthritis.

When I developed arthritis I also noticed that my hands and feet got very cold in cold weather. Is this related to my arthritis?

Patients with a variety of arthritic diseases, especially illnesses such as systemic lupus erythematosus and Sjogren's syndrome, may develop a condition called *Raynaud's phenomenon,* in which there is poor blood flow to the fingers and toes. It also occurs by itself, unassociated with these illnesses. It can be related to the use of vibrating equipment such as jackhammers.

Upon exposure to cold weather, the involved blood vessels constrict or narrow, preventing normal blood flow. The affected fingers and toes become painful and change color. Initially they turn white, then purple, then red. However, all three color changes do not have to be present. Anywhere from one to all of the fingers and toes may be involved. Nervousness may also precipitate attacks. Patients with this problem must be very careful about keeping their bodies warm. In addition, there are some medications that may help the disease, as discussed in Chapter 8.

Finally, we conclude with a discussion of one of the classic old wives' tales in medicine. Or is it?

My joints hurt when the weather changes. Is that my imagination?

This is *not* an old wives' tale! The climate does affect joint symptoms in some patients. Inclement weather usually worsens joint pains, although in some patients it has no effect at all. The reason for this discrepancy is unclear. Patients may also note an increase in the activity of their arthritis when the weather is *changing,* especially when the barometric pressure drops, the humidity rises, and the temperature declines. Thus they feel the effects of a storm before it arrives. Once it does arrive and the above factors stabilize, the increased symptoms may abate. Some patients are so sensitive to these changes that I'm convinced they can predict the weather better than the weather service.

Now you know about the symptoms of arthritis. After taking your medical history, your physician will examine you. The next chapter describes the significance of that examination.

6

Physical Examination of the Patient with Arthritis

The physical examination your doctor performs continues to exert a mystique. We all smile in relief when we're pronounced sound and panic if the doctor frowns while going through the routine. What can be learned from the physical examination? How important is it? These and other questions relating to the examination are answered in this chapter.

What can my doctor tell from examining my joints?

The joint examination can yield a wealth of information that is practical from a diagnostic as well as a therapeutic perspective. The first thing your doctor does when examining your joints is look for evidence of inflammation, such as swelling and redness. This is especially valuable when examining the hands and, to a lesser degree, the feet, areas where joint inflammation is relatively easy to detect. The distribution of arthritic involvement within the hands is a particularly helpful diagnostic tool.

Different arthritic diseases have different appearances. For example, osteoarthritis usually results in growth of new bone around involved joints. This produces a hard, waxy appearance as opposed to the swelling associated with rheumatoid arthritis, which tends to look as if an envelope of fluid were draped around the involved joints. The rheumatoid joint is more likely to have a reddish discoloration than the osteoarthritic joint. The psoriatic joint may have an angry-looking discoloration as well.

The pattern of joint involvement is also important. For example, the small joints at the ends of the fingers are involved in osteoarthritis and psoriatic arthritis but not in rheumatoid arthritis. These joints are called the distal interphalangeal joints. Progressing down the fingers toward the hand, the next finger joint is called the proximal interphalangeal joint. These joints are involved in all forms of arthritis: osteoarthritis, rheumatoid arthritis, and psoriatic arthritis. The next joints, located where the fingers reach the hand, are the metacarpophalangeal joints, or the knuckles. These joints are rarely involved in osteoarthritis but are commonly involved in rheumatoid and psoriatic arthritis.

The examiner then looks at the extent of involvement. Rheumatoid arthritis often involves an entire set of joints, such as all of the knuckles. Osteoarthritis and psoriatic arthritis are spottier in their distribution. Rheumatoid arthritis is also considered a symmetrical disease because similar joints on both sides of the body are usually involved. Thus, if the knuckles of the right hand are involved, most of the knuckles of the left hand will be involved as well. If the right elbow is involved, so is the left. Osteoarthritis may or may not be symmetrical; psoriatic arthritis is usually not.

When all three finger or toe joints are involved in psoriatic arthritis, massive swelling often occurs. This results in a so-called sausage finger or sausage toe, a phenomenon not seen in the other two main types of arthritis.

After inspecting the joints the physician will then gently squeeze them to determine if they are tender. Joints that appear normal may be tender, indicating that they too are involved. Thus the physician continues to map out involved joints, especially in the hands, and a specific picture usually emerges. If all the joints on the ends of the fingers are involved, the patient has osteoarthritis or psoriatic arthritis but not rheumatoid arthritis. Involvement of all the knuckles most likely means rheumatoid arthritis. A spotty, asymmetric distribution involving to some degree all three sets of joints most likely means psoriatic arthritis. Thus, simply by looking at your hands and squeezing the joints, your doctor can often determine the type of arthritis you have. In addition, the physician will feel the joints to determine if they are warm to the touch; warmth indicates the presence of inflammation.

The physician makes an assessment regarding the severity of the arthritis by subjectively determining the degree of swelling, tenderness, and warmth. This is also a helpful way of gauging the patient's response to therapy.

Finally, the physician will move the joints throughout their range of motion to determine if any limitations are present. This indicates which areas need special exercises and strengthening.

Can joint pain be caused by something besides arthritis?

While examining your joints, your doctor is examining areas around the joints as well. For example, a patient may complain of knee pain, but the pain may not actually be coming from the knee. Specific limitations of motion, or tenderness that results from a certain motion, may point to involvement of structures around joints, rather than the joints themselves, as the root of the problem. This is illustrated in the following case history.

Ann Smythe was 56 years old when I saw her in consultation. Her doctor had told her she had arthritis, although he was unsure of the type. When she failed to respond to anti-inflammatory medication, she was referred to me. She complained of pain in a number of areas, specifically the left thumb, right shoulder, left hip, left knee, and right large toe.

Her left thumb looked normal and wasn't tender when I squeezed it. Yet when moved in a certain fashion, it gave her extreme pain. The diagnosis? Not arthritis, but tendinitis of the thumb. As discussed in Chapter 3, *tendons* are strong, elastic bands of tissue that attach muscles to bone. When a muscle contracts, it pulls on its tendon, which then pulls on the connecting bone — that's how our limbs move. When tendons become inflamed, the condition is called *tendinitis*. Examination of Mrs. Smythe's right shoulder revealed certain restrictions of motion accompanied by pain. The diagnosis was also tendinitis.

Mrs. Smythe's left hip and left knee moved normally but were tender over specific areas called bursae. A *bursa* is a saclike structure situated near a joint, sometimes enveloping it. Its main purpose is to protect the joint from surrounding structures such as muscles. Just as tendons can become inflamed, so can bursae. The result is *bursitis*. Mrs. Smythe was suffering from bursitis of the hip and knee, termed trochanteric bursitis and anserine bursitis respectively.

Examination of Mrs. Smythe's toes revealed the presence of a bunion at the base of her right large toe. A *bunion* results when the bursa surrounding a toe becomes enlarged. It is often accompanied by osteoarthritis. Mrs. Smythe's bunion was irritated and painful.

Thus, Mrs. Smythe's main problems were not arthritic in nature. Since tendinitis and bursitis don't always respond to anti-inflammatory medication, she was sent for physical and occupational therapy. She was also sent to a podiatrist, or foot doctor, who fashioned a pad to protect her bunion. After six weeks she was almost entirely pain-free.

In this instance the examination was instrumental in making the correct diagnosis and instituting the appropriate forms of therapy.

Examples of tendinitis and bursitis follow. Many of these conditions have rather interesting names.

Tennis Elbow

This is caused by inflammation and degeneration of the tendons on the outside of the elbow. It is caused by repeated tightening of the muscles of the hand and forearm. Interestingly, only ten percent of people with this problem get it from playing tennis. It also results from twisting tools while using a firm grip or from repeatedly clenching the hands. Politicians may develop this from too much hand-shaking!

Golfer's Elbow

This is similar to tennis elbow, but it is on the inside rather than the outside of the elbow.

Trigger Finger

When the tendons responsible for bending the fingers become inflamed, small nodules may form on them. These often can't pass through the outer lining, or sheath, of the tendon, and movement is blocked.

deQuervain's Tendinitis

This form of tendinitis results from repeated

use of the wrist and the base of the thumb. Although both men and women may develop it, women sometimes develop deQuervain's tendinitis during pregnancy or while caring for newborn babies.

Tailor's Seat

This results from inflammation of the bursa located in the bottom of the pelvis, where we sit. It can make sitting quite painful.

Trochanteric Bursitis

This occurs when the bursa on the outer side of the hip becomes inflamed. It is worsened by pressure, making it uncomfortable to lie on the involved side when sleeping. Pressure on the trochanteric bursa sometimes awakens people from sleep.

Housemaid's Knee

The front of the kneecap is lined by a bursa, which can become inflamed as a result of being subjected to repeated pressure.

Anserine Bursitis

The anserine bursae occur on the inside of

the knees, where they come together. Inflammation most commonly occurs in post-menopausal women with fatty deposits around their knees. Pain is worsened with rest, and sleeping may prove difficult.

The joint examination can therefore be an invaluable aid to your physician. It can help determine the type of arthritis you have and its severity, and differentiate arthritis from other conditions that appear to cause joint pain. But what happens if the joint exam is negative? The answer may surprise you.

My doctor said my examination was normal but I still had arthritis. Is this possible?

It is. The answer to this question illustrates what an inexact science medicine can be. For example, if a patient's history suggests the presence of arthritis — that is, various joints are stiff in the morning upon arising and get better later in the day — the patient probably has joint inflammation, even if the physical examination is normal. Technically, this patient is said to have *arthralgias,* or joint pains without objective evidence of inflammation.

This may sound incongruous. If inflammation is responsible for the discomfort, shouldn't there be proof of its presence? There should be, but the examination may be too insensitive to detect it. If we could routinely use microscopes to look inside normal-looking joints suspected of being arthritic, we would frequently find evidence of inflammation.

There is a test, called *thermography,* that measures the heat emanating from a joint. An inflamed joint gives off more heat than a normal joint, so the test is capable of detecting early inflammation. It's more sensitive than human hands and verifies the thesis that inflammation may be present despite a normal appearance on examination.

By inference we often assume a joint is inflamed by the "company it keeps." If evidence of inflammation, such as swelling, warmth, redness, or tenderness, is present in some joints of a patient with rheumatoid arthritis, it is probably logical to assume that inflammation may also be present in other painful joints, even though they do not display the obvious signs listed above.

Finally, results of the joint exam may depend on when it is performed. We already know there is usually a pattern to a patient's symptoms. In the case of conditions such as rheumatoid arthritis, symptoms are worse upon arising and improve later in the day. The same is true for objective signs of inflammation. If a patient with rheumatoid arthritis has a doctor's appointment at 2:00 in the afternoon, the joint examination may be negative. If the appointment were at 9:00 in the morning, the same exam might be positive. Similarly, osteo-arthritis often worsens as the day progresses and after prolonged activity. Therefore, a joint examination conducted at midmorning might be negative; the same examination after a long afternoon walk could be positive.

The insensitivity of the examination is not unique to the subspecialty of rheumatology. A patient with an ulcer may have a normal abdominal exam. Many of us have heard unfortunate stories of people who went to their physicians complaining of chest pain. Their exams were normal, and more objective tests such as cardiograms were normal as well. Yet they left their doctor's office and had a heart attack. Thankfully, this is a rather rare event. Just as rheumatologists know that a patient with joint complaints may have arthritis despite a negative examination, so cardiologists know that a normal examination does not preclude the possibility of heart disease.

Speaking of hearts leads us to the last question in this section.

My right knee ached — nothing else. Yet my doctor did a complete examination,

including listening to my heart and lungs. Was all this necessary?

Yes, unless perhaps you recently had a complete physical. There are two major reasons for your doctor's compulsive behavior: (1) the need to establish a diagnosis and (2) the need to ascertain your ability to tolerate various types of therapy.

As previously stated, there are over a hundred different types of arthritis, and clues to their presence may be found on physical examination. For example, a thorough inspection of the skin may reveal the presence of psoriasis. Even a small patch of psoriasis, unbeknownst to the patient but discovered on physical examination, may be enough to make the correct diagnosis. Another type of skin rash suggests the diagnosis of Lyme arthritis. A nodule on the forearm may be a *rheumatoid nodule,* which is basically only seen in rheumatoid arthritis. A small nodule on the ear may represent a tophus, or an accumulation of uric acid, the substance responsible for the development of gout. The eyes may be yellow, suggesting the possibility of hepatitis as well as the arthritis that may accompany this condition. A pelvic examination may lead to the diagnosis of a venereal disease, such as gonorrhea, which may be associated with arthritis.

Recently I was asked to see a 49-year-old woman with a two-month history of arthritis. On examination I noted that her nails were shaped in a peculiar fashion, the medical term for which is *clubbing*. The combination of clubbing and a specific type of arthritis is frequently associated with malignancies, especially of the lung. I immediately sent her for a chest x-ray, which revealed the presence of a tumor that turned out to be malignant. On a brighter note, there was no evidence that it had spread. The tumor was surgically removed, and as of this writing the woman is doing well. Possibly, the tumor was discovered in time.

In other words, your doctor looks for a number of things when examining you, including a sense of your general health, as this could impact on your treatment.

In addition, the medications used to treat arthritis have a number of potential side effects. They may lead to fluid retention or blood pressure elevation, especially in a patient who already has these problems. Therefore, your doctor will be particularly interested in your blood pressure, will listen to your lungs to be sure you do not have a buildup of fluid, and will examine the area around your ankles, another potential site of fluid buildup. In fact, fluid retention, called *edema,* must often be differentiated from ankle-swelling caused by arthritis.

Finally, exercise is often part of the treatment for arthritis. Therefore your doctor must assess your physical condition in order to determine what type of exercise program you can tolerate.

Now that you know what your physician is looking for in the physical examination, what about all those fancy laboratory tests that often seem so confusing? Those tests, from the simplest to the most complex, are discussed in the next chapter.

7

Laboratory Tests

Appearances often are deceiving.

— AESOP

Your doctor will probably order a number of laboratory tests to help evaluate your arthritic complaints. These include blood and urine tests, x-rays, and occasionally more sophisticated tests such as CT scans and MRIs. Why are these tests ordered? How are they interpreted? Why do they sometimes have to be repeated? The answers to these and other commonly asked questions about the laboratory investigation of arthritis follow. By the time you have finished this chapter, you will realize why appearances often are deceiving.

Again, we start with the most basic question.

What kind of tests do you order, and why do you order them? Does a rheumatologist order the same tests my family doctor or internist would order?

The laboratory tests used to evaluate the

patient with arthritis fall into two categories — the same tests your regular doctor orders, plus more specific tests for your arthritis. Unless you have recently had routine laboratory tests, such as those usually obtained at the time of a periodic physical, they will most likely be ordered when your arthritis is evaluated. They serve two general purposes — to determine if there are complications of your arthritis and to assess your overall health. Problems with the latter may interfere with treatment, alter treatment, or make it necessary to postpone treatment until an underlying problem is addressed.

The most frequently ordered routine tests are the following.

Complete Blood Count, or CBC

This is a determination of the number of red blood cells you have, their hemoglobin content (hemoglobin is the substance in red blood cells that carries oxygen), and the number of white blood cells present. There is also usually an estimate of the number of platelets present. Platelets are small particles within the blood that help it clot.

The main purpose of a CBC is to determine if you are anemic. *Anemia* is a condition in which the number of red blood cells, or their hemoglobin content, is decreased. Some types of arthritis, such as rheumatoid arthritis, may be associated with anemia — another indication that rheumatoid arthritis is a systemic disease.

The anemia may be a coincidence, in which case its cause must be determined and the condition treated. One of the most common coincidental causes is iron deficiency, a condition particularly common in young women, the same population that is most prone to develop rheumatoid arthritis. The most common explanation for iron deficiency anemia in a woman is menstrual blood loss that is not adequately compensated for by dietary iron intake. However, anemia has a number of other causes and these must be considered before proceeding with therapy. Anemia may also result as a complication of anti-inflammatory drug therapy. These medications may cause inflammation of the lining of the stomach, called gastritis, or an ulcer. Both of these conditions can cause bleeding and lead to anemia.

The CBC can also uncover abnormalities in platelets and the white blood cell count. Again, these abnormalities may be a coincidence or associated with the arthritic disease. A low white blood cell count can be related to rheumatoid arthritis or systemic lupus erythematosus. An unusual complication of rheumatoid arthritis is *Felty's syndrome,* which consists of enlarged lymph nodes and an enlarged spleen (both of which can be detected on physical examination), anemia, and decreased white blood cells and platelets. Paradoxically, an increased platelet count is also associated with rheumatoid arthritis because platelets have a tendency to increase in the presence of severe inflammation. Various medications can also lower the white blood cell and platelet count.

An elevated white blood cell count may be caused by a blood malignancy such as leukemia. A specific type of arthritis is associated with this condition. Thankfully it is rare. Most elevated white blood cell counts are not related to malignancies. Their most common cause is an infection. Another common cause is smoking, which of course is a serious problem as well.

Chemical Profile

This consists of a number of individual tests, the most important of which determine how various organs, such as the liver and kidney, are working. These organs may be involved in various arthritic diseases, most commonly lupus. In addition, since the drugs used to treat arthritis are *metabolized,* or chemically and physically processed by the liver and kidney, these organs must be determined to be functioning normally before long-term therapy is instituted. The tests must also be repeated periodically to be sure problems are not developing in response to therapy. Abnormalities in function may warrant stopping specific medications or lowering their doses.

A uric acid determination is frequently included in the chemical profile. As explained in Chapter 3, deposits of uric acid can crystalize in the joints and cause episodes of gout. Although most patients with gout have elevated uric acid levels, some have normal determinations. In addition, people with increased uric acid levels do not necessarily have gout.

Muscle enzyme tests detect the presence of muscle damage. Various rheumatic diseases are associated with muscle inflammation. This is the primary problem in a disease called *polymyositis,* and it occurs less commonly in a host of other rheumatic illnesses. In fact, minor muscle inflammation may be present in rheumatoid arthritis.

The chemical profile also often includes a determination of the cholesterol level. This is important for everyone but may be especially vital to the arthritis sufferer, who may be inactive, overeat because of depression, and gain weight. As a result, the cholesterol level may rise, potentially causing additional health problems (more on this in Chapter 10).

The various tests in the chemical profile can be ordered on an individual basis as well.

Urinalysis

This encompasses a number of different tests, which reveal the presence of red and white blood cells, protein, sugar, and a variety of substances that should not normally be present in the urine. One of the main functions of this test is to determine how the kidneys are functioning. As noted above, kidney disease may be present in various arthritic diseases, especially lupus. The urinalysis may become abnormal before abnormalities in the blood can be detected by the chemical profile. On the other hand, the chemical profile may be abnormal while the urinalysis is normal — so both tests have to be done.

The urinalysis is also periodically performed to monitor for abnormalities that may develop from therapy with various agents used to treat arthritis, such as anti-inflammatory drugs and gold (see Chapter 8).

On occasion it may become necessary to collect all the urine during a 24-hour period. Not surprisingly, this is called a *24-hour urine collection.* It is ordered when very precise information is needed. For example, a routine urine test may reveal the presence of an abnormal amount of protein in the urine; the 24-hour urine test determines the exact amount. A 24-hour urine test for *creatinine,* which is a normal waste product eliminated by the kidneys, along with a blood creatinine determination, reveals the *creatinine clearance,* a sensitive measure of the kidney's ability to filter waste. As with the chemical profile, abnormalities in the urinalysis may influence the type and dose of medication used.

Hemoccult Test

This is a test to determine occult (hidden) blood in the stool. Significant blood loss in the gastrointestinal tract will result in a black discoloration of the stool, especially when the bleeding occurs in the stomach or beginning of the small intestine. Incidentally, taking iron pills will also turn the stool black. However, you may be losing blood from your gastrointestinal tract without knowing it; that is, your stool may look normal. The only way your physician can determine if you are losing small amounts of blood from your gastrointestinal tract is to test your stool. A stool specimen may be obtained at the time a rectal examination is performed, or your doctor may give you a card to take home. You will then place a small stool sample on the card and send it back to the physician. It is recommended that stool specimens be evaluated routinely, especially in individuals over the age of 40, to facilitate early detection of cancer of the colon. A variety of other conditions can cause blood in the stool, including gastritis, ulcers, and bleeding hemorrhoids.

The stool test for occult blood is particularly valuable to the individual with arthritis. We do not want to administer anti-inflammatory drugs to patients who are bleeding. Anti-inflammatory drugs impair the ability of platelets to function, which may worsen bleeding. As noted, these medications may also result in bleeding by causing gastritis or an ulcer. Thus it is important to recheck the stool periodically after treatment with anti-inflammatory medication has been instituted, even if an earlier test was negative.

The importance of this is graphically illustrated by two of my patients, both men in their late 50s. Both developed positive tests for occult blood in the stool after originally being negative. Coincidentally, both were originally reluctant to undergo further medical tests. Since anti-inflammatory medications may irritate the stomach, both were willing to assume that was the cause of their bleeding. However, I could not assume that was the case and urged both men to have further tests. They ultimately did, and were found to have cancer of the colon. They had surgery, the tumors were removed, and in neither case was there evidence the tumor had spread, so both men have the potential of being cured.

In these two instances the antiplatelet effects of the medications caused the tumors to bleed. In other instances these effects lead to bleeding in previously problem-free hemorrhoids. In still others, gastritis or an ulcer develops, which occurs independently of the antiplatelet effect. In any case, the stool test for occult bleeding is an extremely important, even life-saving test.

If you have had a recent stool test, it is usually unnecessary to obtain another before your therapy begins. If you haven't had a stool test lately, your physician may begin treatment but give you a test card, as described above, and ask that it be promptly returned.

Are there any special laboratory tests for arthritis?

There are indeed a number of rather complicated tests that are often obtained in order to help evaluate a person with joint complaints. For the most part, these sophisticated laboratory tests are used as an adjunct when a physician is faced with making the diagnosis of an arthritic disease. With the exception of the joint fluid analysis, which results in the diagnosis of gout or of an infection, none of them, by themselves, is adequate to make a specific diagnosis.

Erythrocyte Sedimentation Rate

The sed rate, or ESR for short, is a crude index of inflammation; that is, the more inflammation is present, the higher the sed rate. The test is sometimes difficult to interpret, as the sed rate has a tendency to increase with normal aging. The ESR can't differentiate among various types of inflammation. Thus, although rheumatoid arthritis may result in an increased value, so will a host of other diseases such as hepatitis, chronic infections, and ulcerative colitis, to name but a few.

Surprisingly, the test may be normal despite the presence of an inflammatory condition. I vividly recall a patient a colleague of mine at Harvard asked me to see. This woman had all the symptoms of rheumatoid arthritis, and her physical examination strongly suggested this diagnosis as well. When I asked him why he questioned the diagnosis, he asked how she could have rheumatoid arthritis with a normal sedimentation rate. Although I couldn't tell him why the sedimentation rate had not increased, I assured him the situation was not unusual.

On the other hand, some patients with illnesses such as rheumatoid arthritis and lupus have sedimentation rates that rise and fall in concert with the activity of the disease. In such a situation, this test may be a helpful way of assessing a patient's response to therapy.

Rheumatoid Factor

This is an autoantibody (see Chapter 4) directed against a specific normal factor in the patient's blood. The test got its name because the autoantibody is often present in patients with rheumatoid arthritis, but it is only present in seventy-five to eighty percent of these patients. It takes time for the test to become positive. It is negative in fifty percent of individuals who have had rheumatoid arthritis for less than six months.

Like the sedimentation rate, the rheumatoid factor is often a source of confusion. *A patient can have rheumatoid arthritis in the face of a negative test.* This may be because the test has not yet had a chance to become positive or because the patient being tested is one of the twenty to twenty-five percent who test negative in any case. The situation is further complicated by the fact that a number of diseases other than rheumatoid arthritis are associated with positive tests. In addition, some normal individuals test positive. The incidence of positive tests in normal people increases with the age of the person being tested. Therefore, a positive test alone is insufficient to make the diagnosis of rheumatoid arthritis.

When patients ask if arthritis shows up in the blood, they are usually referring to the rheumatoid factor as well as the test that follows, the antinuclear antibody.

Antinuclear antibody

Like the rheumatoid factor, this is an antibody, or more specifically a group of antibodies, directed against the nuclei of one's own cells. Although present in the vast majority of patients with systemic lupus erythematosus, it is also present in patients with a host of other diseases, including rheumatoid arthritis. Also, like the rheumatoid factor, this test can be positive in normal individuals, especially as they grow older. The test is helpful in ascertaining the diagnosis of lupus only if a number of other classical criteria are present. *A positive test is insufficient to make the diagnosis of SLE unless other criteria are present.*

HLA B 27 Antigen

This is a gene that is detected by a blood test. As discussed in Chapter 4, the gene is present in approximately ninety percent of patients with ankylosing spondylitis, so some physicians use its presence to make this diagnosis. However, the gene is also present in approximately eight percent of the white population and four percent of the black population. Thus its presence may be a coincidence and does not necessarily confirm the diagnosis of ankylosing spondylitis.

Test for Lyme Disease

This blood test may be falsely negative early after the tick bite. It may be falsely positive in healthy individuals and in those with a variety of other diseases. Finally, a small group of people who have been infected by the organism that causes Lyme disease do not have symptoms but test positive. If they have symptoms caused by another illness, those symptoms may be mistakenly attributed to Lyme disease.

Joint Fluid Analysis

It is sometimes necessary to remove, or

aspirate, fluid from a joint. Joint fluid is also called synovial fluid, a certain amount of which is normally present. Various forms of arthritis result in increased production of synovial fluid. Analysis of the fluid sometimes yields very important information. It may enable your doctor to make the specific diagnosis of gout or of an infection.

My tests were negative, but my doctor told me I still had arthritis. How can that be?

Since there is a great deal of confusion regarding the interpretation of laboratory tests, this point deserves emphasis. Just as a positive blood test does not confirm the diagnosis of an arthritic disease, a negative test does not rule it out. As noted above, it is possible to have rheumatoid arthritis with a negative rheumatoid factor, ankylosing spondylitis without the HLA B 27 gene, and active arthritis of any type with a normal sedimentation rate. You may even have gout with a normal uric acid level. It is unlikely for someone to have lupus with a negative antinuclear antibody test but, to repeat, a positive ANA does not necessarily mean you have lupus.

You already did the tests once. Why do they have to be repeated?

Reasons vary from test to test. Sometimes the sedimentation rate waxes and wanes with disease activity. If this is the case it can be a useful measure for gauging your response to therapy. The rheumatoid factor may take as long as two years, or longer in the atypical patient, to turn positive. Your physician may therefore check it periodically within the first two years but seldom thereafter. The antinuclear antibody, as well as similar but more sophisticated tests such as that for anti-double-stranded DNA antibodies (which is a more specific test for SLE), may also fluctuate with disease activity. Should this not be the case, it seldom makes sense to repeat the tests.

The routine tests, such as the CBC, chemical profile, urinalysis, and stool test for occult blood, are repeated on a more regular basis to be sure the patient is not developing any complications from the disease or the medication (more on the complications of medication in the next chapter).

Some of the more sophisticated tests do not have to be repeated. For example, there is no need to repeat the HLA B 27 antigen. As noted, the HLA B 27 is a gene. Since genes do not change — you always have the same genes — there is no reason to repeat this test. The rare exception would be if your doctor thought there was a laboratory error.

$$\star \; \star \; \star$$

In addition to the tests discussed above, doctors often utilize x-rays to help evaluate patients with joint complaints. A number of questions surround the use of these and similar but more sophisticated diagnostic tests.

What can my doctor tell from x-rays?

X-rays offer objective proof that arthritis is present and help differentiate among the types. The x-ray images of rheumatoid arthritis and osteoarthritis are usually quite different. Rheumatoid arthritis is characterized by the presence of *erosions,* or holes in the bone. In addition, the bones around the rheumatoid joint often appear thin, or less dense than normal. Thinning of bones, in general, is referred to as *osteoporosis.* Typically, osteoporosis occurs in the wrists, low back or lumbar spine, and hips. When it occurs in association with rheumatoid arthritis, the formal medical term is *juxta articular osteopenia,* or thinning of the bone around the joint. The x-ray findings of psoriatic arthritis and gout are somewhat similar to those of rheumatoid arthritis, although juxta articular bone loss is less of a feature.

Osteoarthritis is characterized by narrowing of the joint space, or the space separating the two bones forming the joint. As previously noted, osteoarthritis is primarily a disease of cartilage, or the tissue that lines the ends of the bones forming a joint. Cartilage does not show up on an x-ray; the beam simply passes through it without leaving an image on the film. Cartilage appears on the x-ray as a space separating adjoining bones. If the cartilage becomes narrowed, that space decreases. Thus, if your doctor tells you your joint space is narrowed, what this really means is that the amount of cartilage is diminished.

The presence of osteoarthritis on x-rays is not necessarily a cause for concern. Many people over the age of 60 display x-ray evidence of osteoarthritis, yet few have symptoms of the disease. Therefore, the presence of osteoarthritis on an x-ray does not prove the patient's pain is associated with that finding — it may simply be a coincidence. To make matters more complicated, osteoarthritis can develop in a joint originally afflicted by rheumatoid or psoriatic arthritis.

From a diagnostic perspective, x-rays not only help differentiate among the various types of arthritis but may also identify the presence of conditions such as tendinitis and bursitis. X-rays also offer a way to measure the severity of the arthritis objectively and to follow the progress of the disease and its response to therapy. For example, by counting the number of erosions present before and after administration of a specific medication to a patient with rheumatoid arthritis, the effectiveness of that drug can be determined.

It seems that x-rays are an invaluable tool. But is that always so? This issue is addressed in the next question.

I went to the doctor because of shoulder pain and my doctor treated me without taking an x-ray. Shouldn't an x-ray have been ordered?

X-rays are not always necessary. Your physician can often make a diagnosis based on your history and physical examination. Your response to therapy then determines if further evaluation is indicated. In the specific question above, the physician may have made the diagnosis of tendinitis and instituted the appropriate therapy. Assuming the therapy is successful, there is no need to obtain an x-ray. On the other hand, if the doctor had doubts or if the response to treatment was less than optimal, an x-ray would be ordered.

Similarly, since osteoarthritis of the hands is often a relatively easy diagnosis to make, x-rays may be unnecessary, especially initially.

Should the patient not do well, x-rays would probably be ordered to be certain another type of arthritis was not present and to determine the extent of the osteoarthritis.

Is there a reason *not* to order an x-ray?

The answer is twofold. First, x-rays obviously expose the patient to radiation. Although radiation exposure resulting from a single set of joint films is minimal, the effects of radiation are cumulative. In addition, x-rays cost money, whether the patient, an insurance company, or the government winds up paying for them. In other words, they should always be ordered with a purpose in mind.

The next two questions emphasize points previously made. Both are very frequently asked.

My x-rays are negative. Does that mean I don't have arthritis?

Not necessarily. Just as you can have arthritis with negative blood tests, you can have arthritis with normal x-rays. It takes time — months or even years — for the changes to occur that show up on an x-ray. That is another reason why some physicians may not order x-rays when initially evaluating a patient — it may simply be too early for x-ray abnormalities to be present.

Similarly, it is also possible to have a number of other conditions, such as tendinitis and bursitis, with normal x-rays.

My doctor said the x-rays of my hands show I have osteoporosis. Does that mean I have osteoporosis in other areas? My grandmother has osteoporosis and broke her hip. Will the same thing happen to me?

As noted above, the occurrence of bone thinning around a rheumatoid joint is referred to as juxta articular osteopenia. It is a localized form of osteoporosis and has no relationship to osteoporosis elsewhere. In other words, there is no increased risk of bone fracture in areas such as the hip and back. It should be noted, however, that inactivity is a risk factor for the development of osteoporosis. Thus patients with arthritis whose activities are limited are at increased risk for developing this potentially disabling bone problem.

Finally, what about newer technology? Modern diagnostic tools have a number of applications, as noted in the following questions.

My doctor thought my knee pain wasn't coming from arthritis and ordered an MRI. What is that?

MRI stands for *magnetic resonance imaging.* Simply put, this machine uses magnetic waves, which a computer analyzes to form pictures of various parts of the body.

An x-ray cannot show the nonbony structures, or so-called soft tissues, around joints: tendons, ligaments, and menisci. *Menisci* are structures within joints that help stabilize them. Although made of cartilage, they are not to be confused with *articular cartilage,* which, as discussed previously, covers the ends of the bones that form a joint.

When someone says they tore a cartilage, they really mean they tore a meniscus. This, and similar injuries to tendons and ligaments, can be diagnosed by obtaining an MRI.

For the most part the MRI has replaced a test called an *arthrogram.* An arthrogram is obtained by injecting dye into the joint being studied and taking an x-ray. The dye outlines structures such as menisci, thus enabling abnormalities to be detected.

In addition to being an excellent tool for detecting tendon and ligament abnormalities, MRIs are also used to evaluate possible disc problems in the neck and back.

Another test that yields information similar to the MRI is called *computerized tomography,* or CT scan for short. It is a sophisticated x-ray machine, which provides us with much more detail than standard x-rays. The CT scan is probably superior to the MRI for detecting subtle bone abnormalities but inferior for detecting soft tissue problems. Unlike MRI testing, CT scans result in radiation exposure. Both tests are performed within a small, confined space. The closed-in feeling bothers a few patients, and claustrophobic people are sometimes incapable of completing the test. Obese people sometimes can't fit into the machines.

My doctor thought I had osteoporosis and ordered a CT scan — why not just an x-ray?

Although x-rays have classically been used to detect the presence of osteoporosis, they are poor diagnostic tools because of their relative insensitivity. In fact, *at least 30 percent of bone mass must be lost before osteoporosis is visible on x-rays.* Once it is visible on x-rays it is usually rather advanced. Therefore, a normal x-ray does not rule out the presence of osteoporosis. Thankfully, there are two modern diagnostic tests that are much more sensitive than standard x-rays, namely quantitative computerized tomography, and *dual photon absorptiometry*. Both utilize x-ray beams to measure the density of the bone, but dual photon absorptiometry exposes the patient to less radiation.

CT scans are relatively expensive and can only be applied to the back. Thus the other major area at risk, the hip, cannot be reliably assessed by CT scans. Dual photon absorptiometry is less expensive than computerized tomography and can be applied to the hip as well as the back.

The final diagnostic test available to evaluate osteoporosis is *single photon absorptiometry*, which can only detect osteoporosis in the wrist, the third major site in the body susceptible to the development of osteoporosis. This is the least expensive of the three tests.

It was once thought that the presence of osteoporosis in the wrist indicated similar involvement of the back and hip. This is not true. Although some have advocated single photon absorptiometry as a screening test for osteoporosis of the back and hip, it is too unreliable to have any practical value.

It was also thought that osteoporosis in the back reflected the presence of osteoporosis in the hip. This also is not true. If you undergo either CT scanning or dual photon absorptiometry of the back, and the test is normal, it does not mean your hip is normal. Similarly, if the tests are abnormal, it does not necessarily mean the hip is abnormal as well. In other words, each area must be individually evaluated.

It is not generally recommended that these tests be used to screen people for osteoporosis. You have a greater than average risk of developing osteoporosis if you are a woman (white women are at greatest risk, followed by Asians; Hispanics and blacks are at lowest risk) with a family history of osteoporosis or with a low body weight; had an early menopause (before the age of 45); have been on long-term steroid therapy; or have abnormalities of calcium metabolism. If you fit into any of these categories, discuss bone density testing with your doctor. Other factors that increase your risk of developing osteoporosis include a low intake of calcium-containing foods, a sedentary lifestyle, and regular use of alcohol, cigarettes, and coffee.

My doctor ordered an ultrasound test of my knee. What is it, and what can it tell?

In *diagnostic ultrasound,* sound waves are bounced off a structure in order to obtain information about that structure. It is similar in principle to the use of sonar. An ultrasound of the knee is usually performed to detect the presence of a *Baker's cyst*. This is a swelling located behind the knee and is actually an extension, or herniation, of the knee joint. On occasion Baker's cysts rupture, leading to swelling of the calf.

The final question in this chapter is usually the most frightening.

My doctor wants to do a biopsy of my knee. Does that mean I may have cancer?

A biopsy is the removal of a small piece of tissue from your body. The specimen is usually viewed under a microscope, but it can be subjected to a number of other tests as well. It is rarely necessary to perform joint biopsies. When they are done, it is usually to help determine the type of arthritis present. Cancer of the joint is quite rare.

You can see why the quote that began this chapter, "Appearances often are deceiving," is appropriate. You can have arthritis with negative lab tests, and positive lab tests don't necessarily mean a thing. The tests must be interpreted in light of your history and physical examination. By themselves they are often meaningless.

★ ★ ★

Now that we know what arthritis is and how it is evaluated, let's discuss its treatment. The next chapter is the first of three dealing with this very important topic.

8

Medications

There is perhaps no misconception more pervasive than the one that nothing can be done to treat arthritis. Nothing could be further from the truth. The treatment program is comprehensive. It is basically a three-pronged affair consisting of medication, physical therapy, and an overall conditioning program. Added to this are measures to control your diet, ensure adequate rest, and reduce stress to the greatest possible degree.

This chapter is about the medications used to treat arthritis — their indications, their relative dangers, how they interact with other drugs, and a number of other issues that come up on an almost daily basis. Additional aspects of therapy are addressed in subsequent chapters.

The benefits to be gained by treating arthritis with medication are illustrated by continuing Mickey Mantle's story. As noted in Chapter 2, Mantle had to retire prematurely because of arthritis in both knees. At first he attributed the discomfort to his age. When he discovered he had osteoarthritis, he tried over-the-counter medications without success. He thought nothing could be done to treat arthritis.

As the pain worsened he became more and more depressed. He rarely played golf, one of his two favorite sports. Golf was more than a game, it was almost a way of life. It was the way he kept fit, the way he fulfilled his competitive needs, the way he socialized. He reached the point where he rarely played. He still went to the golf course but didn't participate, just watched his friends.

In 1987 he was treated with an anti-inflammatory drug, which, as he put it, "brightened my life." The pain and discomfort decreased, his knees became more flexible, he had less trouble with stairs, and he even returned to playing golf regularly. In fact, his knees used to swell by the end of the day even when he was relatively inactive. After being treated with an anti-inflammatory drug they don't swell after eighteen holes of golf.

Mantle's experience is not a miracle. There are no miracles in medicine. But his story does illustrate how much people can improve when given the proper treatment.

Mantle's teammate and friend Whitey Ford tells a similar story. Also an avid golfer, Ford and his wife went on a golfing vacation to Ireland. Accustomed to using a golf cart, they walked the courses because none was available. He walked more during that two-week period than he had in years. He soon developed left knee pain, and when it didn't go away sought medical care. An x-ray revealed the presence of arthritis. He was surprised because he never had knee problems as a player. He also thought he was too young to develop arthritis.

His activities became limited. He had pitched batting practice in spring training for the Yankees. Now he couldn't. He and Mantle have a baseball camp for adults in Florida, the Mantle Ford Fantasy Camp. He had pitched to the campers. Now he couldn't. He had played golf on a regular basis, sometimes daily. In the year after he developed arthritis he only played two rounds of golf. He had liked to walk on the beach. He reached the point where he walked as little as possible.

In his own words, he was "down in the dumps."

A conversation with Mantle's wife inspired Ford to seek appropriate care. She told him how well Mickey was doing, and soon thereafter Ford saw a physician who treated him with an anti-inflammatory drug. He had an excellent response. He returned to golf, often playing four times a week, he again pitched batting practice for the Yankees during spring training, and he resumed an active role in his baseball camp, pitching to both sides during a nine-inning game.

These are not isolated stories. Thousands of people benefit from various types of medication to treat arthritis. In order for you to benefit, you should know as much about them as possible.

I can put up with the pain. Why treat it?

As I often tell my patients, life isn't an endurance contest — at least it shouldn't be. It's not normal to have pain, and no one should have to live with it. In addition, pain tells us something is wrong, and that information shouldn't be ignored. Pain should be used as a gauge, an indicator of an underlying problem.

In addition to relieving discomfort, it is important to treat arthritic pain because it often correlates with inflammation, and inflammation can damage joints. Furthermore, patients with arthritis have a tendency to *splint* their joints, or not move them through their full range of motion. It's just too painful to do so. Even when patients think they are moving their joints normally, they usually are not.

The unconscious mind is quick to detect even minor pain and anticipate when it will occur. It then sends a message to the involved joint that says, in essence, "Don't move any further." The ultimate result is scarring of the joint and a loss of motion. The muscles around the joint also begin to weaken, or *atrophy*, with lack of normal use, and this ultimately leads to additional motion loss.

Minimizing inflammation and pain makes it easier to maintain normal joint motion as well as muscle tone around the joint. Thus some of the potential damage is reduced or eliminated. Medications alone may not be able to accomplish this. Other types of treatment, such as physical therapy, may also be necessary.

Why can't I just take an over-the-counter medication, like Tylenol® or Nuprin®?

People with arthritis who treat themselves with over-the-counter preparations may be doing themselves a disservice.

Tylenol® is the most common brand name for the drug *acetaminophen.* It is marketed under a number of other brand names, including Anacin-3®, Datril®, and Panadol®. Acetaminophen is an analgesic, which means it reduces pain. It is also an antipyretic, which means it reduces fever. However, acetamino-phen *is not an anti-inflammatory drug.* It may reduce the pain, but not the inflammation of arthritis. An advantage of acetaminophen is that it is rarely associated with side effects. It does not cause an upset stomach and does not cause ulcers. On the other hand, it can't be taken in large doses over a prolonged period of time with impunity, as it has been known to affect the liver.

Advil®, Nuprin®, and Medipren® contain 200 mg of *ibuprofen,* an anti-inflammatory drug, which at higher doses requires a pre-scription. A single 200-mg dose of ibuprofen is sufficient to serve as an analgesic, but it does not significantly reduce inflammation. It is recommended that the daily dose of over-the-counter ibuprofen not exceed 1200 mg. It is at this dose that a mild anti-inflammatory effect may begin to be noted. Over-the-counter ibuprofen can upset the stomach and should always be taken with food or milk. See below for a list of side effects associated with ibu-profen. These occur less often at the over-the-counter dose.

Always tell your physician if you are taking over-the-counter medications. It is not a good idea to mix over-the-counter ibuprofen with a prescription anti-inflammatory drug. Taking an anti-inflammatory drug called diflunisal

(Dolobid®) when you're also taking acetaminophen may cause elevated blood levels of
acetaminophen.

For the most part, these medications
are pain relievers or at best mild anti-
inflammatory drugs. They should be used
under specific circumstances. A patient with
mild osteoarthritis may be quite comfortable
on one of these medications. But unless there
are specific medical reasons to avoid standard
anti-inflammatory drugs, arthritic pain should
generally be treated with anti-inflammatory
medications, not analgesics.

When I explain these concepts to patients,
I often use as an example a 56-year-old man
I saw when I was an intern. Frederick Smith
hated taking medication, but he hated going
to doctors even more. So when he developed
chest pain he simply went to his corner pharmacy and bought some Tylenol®. Being an
active man, he thought he had pulled a muscle,
and the Tylenol® did indeed lessen the pain.
It was only when he developed a high fever
a few days later that he went to the hospital,
where he was found to have pneumonia.
Thankfully, after a course of antibiotics, Mr.
Smith was as good as new.

Even though he had pneumonia all along,
acetaminophen initially made him feel better.
Yet the specific treatment for Mr. Smith's

pneumonia was antibiotics. Similarly, analgesics make arthritis pain better — but the specific treatment is usually anti-inflammatory medication.

My doctor said to take aspirin. What good will that do?

In fact, it may do a lot of good. Historically, aspirin has been the mainstay of arthritis treatment. It became commercially available in 1899. Like ibuprofen, aspirin is an analgesic in low doses but in higher doses an anti-inflammatory drug. What constitutes a higher dose? The initial anti-inflammatory aspirin dose is usually 8 tablets per day (the standard aspirin tablet contains 325 mg, or 5 grains, of acetylsalicylate), and the dose is increased until the patient achieves significant improvement or until side effects occur, whichever comes first. There are prescription aspirin preparations, such as Easprin® and Zorprin®, which contain high doses of aspirin and therefore require fewer pills per day. Easprin® is an enteric-coated tablet (see below) that contains 975 mg of aspirin and is taken three to four times per day. Zorprin® contains 800 mg of aspirin in a time-release capsule designed to be taken twice a day. Some physicians monitor aspirin levels in the blood and discontinue the drug if arbitrary levels are reached without improvement in the arthritis. Before the advent of the newer drugs described below, I saw patients who were taking as many as thirty-two aspirin tablets a day!

A number of aspirin derivatives are available on a prescription basis. Many consider them safer than high doses of standard aspirin, but some doubt they are as effective as other anti-inflammatory drugs. Examples of these medications are salsalate (Disalcid®) and choline magnesium trisalicylate (Trilisate®).

It is not unusual for side effects to occur as a result of aspirin therapy, especially at the doses used to treat arthritis.

What are aspirin's side effects?

Aspirin has many potential side effects. Only the most common will be discussed here.

Gastrointestinal Effects

This refers to problems that develop within the digestive tract, most commonly in the stomach. Typical symptoms include heartburn, abdominal pain, and nausea. Some people say their stomach "just doesn't feel right." More serious complications include the development of *gastritis*, which is the medical term for inflammation of the stomach, and ulcers. Both of these conditions can cause bleeding.

A number of aspirin products contain an antacid to protect the stomach. These probably do not significantly decrease the number of major gastrointestinal problems associated with aspirin. Enteric-coated aspirin does not dissolve until it reaches the small intestine and probably is associated with a reduced number of stomach upsets, but it takes a relatively long time for coated aspirin to be absorbed into your system. Many people find it inadequate if they desire quick pain relief.

Effects on Hearing

Aspirin causes a high-pitched ringing in the ear called *tinnitus*. Some individuals also develop decreased hearing, dizziness, and loss of balance. These side effects are *dose-related;* that is, the higher the dose, the more likely they will occur. In fact, anyone who takes enough aspirin would eventually develop tinnitus and decreased hearing. Older patients are more likely to develop these problems than younger individuals.

Effects on Blood Clotting

Aspirin interferes with platelets, which, as

mentioned in Chapter 6, are small particles in the blood that help it clot. This rarely leads to complications unless there are related problems. For example, bleeding from cuts may take longer to clot, and bleeding associated with gastritis may be more severe than it would be otherwise. This effect lasts for ten to fourteen days after the aspirin has been stopped. Aspirin should be stopped approximately two weeks before surgery in order to avoid excessive bleeding.

Aspirin's ability to decrease the effectiveness of platelets can also be a plus in helping to prevent major problems such as heart attacks and strokes, which may be at least partially caused by the development of clots.

Effects on the Liver

Aspirin sometimes causes liver inflammation, which is usually minor and disappears when the drug is stopped.

Allergic Reactions

These are of two basic types. Some patients may develop asthma after taking aspirin, a risk that is increased in people who have polyps in their noses. The second type of reaction produces a type of skin rash and swelling called *urticaria* and *angioedema* respectively. If you have a history of allergic reactions to aspirin, be sure to tell your doctor. Also, do not take any kind of medication, even over-the-counter preparations such as ibuprofen, without first discussing it with your physician.

Are there alternatives to aspirin?

As noted, in high doses aspirin reduces inflammation. A number of other drugs reduce inflammation as well. These medications are collectively termed *nonsteroidal anti-inflammatory drugs*. This term is used to differentiate these medications from steroids, often referred to as cortisone. Generally, these medications are easier to administer and have less frequent gastrointestinal side effects than high doses of aspirin. It therefore comes as no great surprise that fewer and fewer physicians routinely use aspirin to treat arthritis.

The various anti-inflammatory drugs, along with the pill sizes available and the average dose range, are listed in the table at the end of the chapter. The medications are listed in alphabetical order by their chemical (generic) names followed by the brand name.

The dose ranges listed are averages. Your doctor may ask you to take a higher or lower dose. Never change the dose on your own, even if your

dose is less than the average doses noted here.
Given the number of anti-inflammatory drugs available, the following is a very logical question.

How do I know my doctor is giving me the right drug? How does the doctor choose a specific anti-inflammatory drug?

Physicians choose drugs on the basis of their own experiences, articles in the medical literature, lectures they've attended, and comments and opinions of respected colleagues. Unfortunately, not every medication works for everyone, and your physician employs a trial-and-error approach in order to determine what is best for you. This may sound less than scientific, but there is reason for encouragement — the majority of patients with arthritis are ultimately very pleased with their care.

There is also significant precedent for this type of approach. For example, when treating high blood pressure, physicians may make a number of changes before discovering the most appropriate regimen for a given individual.

Is it always smooth sailing once the most appropriate medication is started? This concern is reflected in the next question, and the answer presents an extremely important concept.

I was doing well on my medication for a number of months, and then my arthritis flared. Why is that? Did I become immune to the medication? If I have to keep changing medications, do you doctors know what you're doing?

Arthritis is an unpredictable disease whose course frequently changes. No one knows what causes it to flare after having been well controlled for a period of time. Similarly, no one knows why a medication that is initially successful loses its effectiveness. A medication may be effective indefinitely in certain people. The same drug given to similar people with the same problem may prove worthless. Again, we don't yet have an explanation for this. So if doctors have to change drugs occasionally, it doesn't mean they don't know what they're doing. It's just a reflection of the variable nature of the disease.

Can anti-inflammatory drugs improve morning stiffness?

As discussed in Chapter 5, morning stiffness is a common complaint among patients with arthritis. It is especially severe in individuals with inflammatory diseases like rheumatoid arthritis.

Tell your doctor if your morning stiffness continues to be a problem; it is often an indication that your arthritis is inadequately controlled. Your physician may want to increase the dose of your anti-inflammatory drug. If you are already receiving the maximum allowable dose of your medication, your doctor may consider switching you to one of the longer-acting agents. For example, if you are on a drug taken three or four times per day, you may be switched to one taken only once or twice daily. Piroxicam (Feldene®) is presently the only anti-inflammatory drug taken on a once-a-day basis. A number of other medications, including diclofenac (Voltaren®), diflunisal (Dolobid®), flurbiprofen (Ansaid®), naproxen (Naprosyn®), and sulindac (Clinoril®), are administered twice daily. Since these drugs remain in the bloodstream for relatively long periods of time, they may still be present after a night's sleep and thus be available to control inflammation and morning stiffness.

Unfortunately, there is often a gap between theory and practice. Thus morning stiffness may remain a problem even with the previously mentioned medications. An alteration in the way the medications are taken may prove productive. For example, piroxicam is often taken after breakfast. This can be changed to either after dinner or before going to sleep, taken with milk, an antacid, or a small snack. The medications taken twice a day are usually taken after breakfast and dinner. The latter dose can be moved to before going to sleep.

If none of these tactics work, try setting your alarm clock for a half hour to an hour before you usually get up. Keep some food or a thermos full of milk handy and take your anti-inflammatory medication. Rest or go back to sleep if you can. Get up at your usual time, and your stiffness may be much better than usual.

Do anti-inflammatory drugs have side effects?

Like most medications, anti-inflammatory drugs can produce a number of side effects. These are categorized as follows.

Gastrointestinal Effects

The most frequently encountered side effects are an upset stomach, indigestion, abdominal discomfort, heartburn, nausea, decreased appetite, diarrhea or constipation, and *stomatitis,* which is the medical term for inflammation or ulcers of the mouth. The above symptoms usually occur within the first days to weeks of therapy, but they can occur at any time. These agents are generally less irritating to the gastrointestinal tract than large anti-inflammatory doses of aspirin.

More serious gastrointestinal complications, such as bleeding (usually from gastritis or an ulcer) and perforation of an ulcer, occur less commonly. *These problems may occur at any time with or without the prior development of symptoms.* If you develop severe abdominal pain, vomit blood, pass black-colored stool (which indicates the presence of blood), or feel dizzy or weak, especially when going from the lying to the sitting or standing position (which may indicate loss of blood), please call your doctor immediately.

Liver Effects

Like aspirin, anti-inflammatory drugs may result in liver disease. This is almost always mild and disappears when the medication is stopped. Rarely, more serious problems develop. Although any anti-inflammatory drug may injure the liver, diclofenac (Voltaren®) and sulindac (Clinoril®) are more likely than the others to do so. Phenylbutazone has been associated with some of the more serious cases of liver damage.

Effects on Blood Clotting

Like aspirin, nonsteroidal anti-inflammatory drugs inhibit the effectiveness of platelets. This effect is shorter-lived than with aspirin and disappears when the drug is gone from the body, which is usually in a matter of days.

Kidney Effects

Although anti-inflammatory medications may have a number of diverse effects on the kidney, these fall into two general categories. First, these drugs may interfere with the kidney's ability to filter the blood. This seldom occurs unless underlying problems, such as heart failure, liver disease, or pre-existing kidney disease, are present. The use of diuretics, or "water pills," may increase the risk of kidney problems. Once the anti-inflammatory drug is stopped, the adverse effects usually disappear.

In addition, anti-inflammatory drugs may directly damage the kidney. Although all the drugs in this class may cause kidney disease, the greatest number of cases have been reported with fenoprofen (Nalfon®). Although the problem usually corrects itself once the drug is withdrawn, this may take months, or even years.

Effects on Blood Pressure

This is rarely a problem unless the patient has pre-existing hypertension or increased blood pressure. Under those circumstances the addition of an anti-inflammatory drug may further elevate the blood pressure and make its control more difficult.

Fluid Retention

This can be a serious problem, especially in an individual who also has a heart problem. The majority of patients who develop this problem say they feel bloated. Others notice swelling, especially in their ankles.

Other Effects

Anti-inflammatory medications may be associated with a plethora of other side effects, including rashes; allergic reactions similar to those described above with aspirin; anemia and decreased white blood cell counts, which are more commonly seen with phenyl-butazone, especially in women over the age of 60; dizziness; fatigue; headaches, especially with indomethacin; blurry vision; and confusion, which occurs more often in the elderly, especially those treated with indomethacin.

Should these or any other problems arise while taking anti-inflammatory drugs, call your doctor.

Do not assume a side effect is "acceptable" or "supposed to happen." The development of such a problem is usually an indication to stop the drug or take other measures to counteract the problem. Once informed of possible side effects, some people erroneously assume that since they are "expected," there is nothing to be done should they occur. This is not the case with anti-inflammatory drugs, but confusion exists because it is the case with some other medications, especially anticancer drugs. Some anticancer drugs result in nausea *every* time they are taken; others universally depress the white blood cell count; others always make you lose your hair. Under these circumstances, the side effects must be accepted. Such is not the case with the drugs used to treat arthritis.

When patients are informed of the potential side effects of anti-inflammatory drugs, the next question usually follows.

It sounds as if anti-inflammatory drugs are dangerous. Is it really worth the risk of taking them?

Physicians have an obligation to be as honest

with their patients as possible, to take the time to educate them about their diseases and their treatments. Any time the patient is started on a new drug, a discussion of its possible side effects is essential. Only when patients are armed with this information can they recognize early side effects so that corrective action can be taken.

Although I've always felt strongly about this, its importance hit home the hard way. My father almost died from a side effect of a drug used to treat his heart condition. When he was recovering I asked him if his physician had warned him about potential complications and was shocked to learn that this had not been done. Ironically, my dad had asked his doctor if potential problems were associated with his new drug. His doctor had responded that he didn't want to give him anything to worry about. As it turned out, my father experienced minor problems for a few days before the situation critically worsened. The particular side effect he developed was a common one, one most physicians would discuss with their patients. If he had been properly educated, the drug would have been stopped immediately, sparing him a potentially life-threatening situation.

There's no substitute for education. Of course it is difficult for the patient to weigh the pluses of anti-inflammatory drugs against their minuses. The list of potential problems is indeed an imposing one. Yet these complications, especially the more serious ones, occur relatively infrequently. With proper patient education, careful monitoring, and the judicious use of various medications to prevent and treat the more common complications, such as gastrointestinal problems, the incidence and severity of side effects can be minimized.

On the other side of the coin, anti-inflammatory drugs can be enormously beneficial. A doctor who has made the decision to use such a medication has made the calculation that the benefits far outweigh the risks.

Perhaps the best way of putting this into perspective is to state that if I had arthritis I would not hesitate to take an anti-inflammatory drug.

Once I'm on an anti-inflammatory drug, what can I do to maximize safety?

Since the most common side effects of these drugs involve the gastrointestinal system, especially the stomach, they should *always* be taken after meals. Food serves as a buffer, thus at least partially protecting the stomach. *If you don't eat, don't take the drug.*

People often ask how much they should eat. As a generalization, there is no need to alter one's normal eating habits. If routine meals are insufficient to protect the stomach, it's seldom worthwhile to add food. One exception is the breakfast that consists of only orange juice and black coffee. That combination can cause an upset stomach even in someone who is not taking an anti-inflammatory drug! A well-balanced meal, with the addition of cereal or an occasional egg, is preferable.

Some medications must be taken four times a day, which is often an inconvenience. These medications are best taken after meals and before going to bed, the latter with a light snack. Thus this particular dose regimen may be responsible for adding calories to one's diet, a distinct disadvantage to most arthritis sufferers.

Are there any foods or medicines that should be avoided while on anti-inflammatory medication?

The prime substance that should be consumed with caution while on anti-inflammatory medication is alcohol, which is of course itself a drug. Alcohol by itself can cause bleeding from the gastrointestinal tract and appears to increase the gastrointestinal side effects associated with anti-inflammatory drugs.

When patients of mine start taking anti-inflammatory drugs, I suggest they abstain from alcohol until it is determined that they can tolerate the medication. Thereafter, I tell them, it's probably OK to resume alcohol, but in moderation and not on a regular basis. Also, it is wise to separate the alcohol from the medication by at least a few hours. When my patients tell me they want to "celebrate" and have more than one or two drinks, I tell them to skip a few doses of their medication that day. Although this is not completely fool-proof, it appears to be reasonably effective in reducing gastrointestinal problems.

In addition to alcohol, patients should be wary of foods that they know routinely give them indigestion. A particular patient comes to mind. He loves pizza, but every time he eats pizza he gets heartburn. When he was placed on an anti-inflammatory medication, the heartburn increased significantly. It disappeared when he stopped eating pizza.

Finally, some medications may create problems when taken along with anti-inflammatory drugs; for example, various oral medications used to treat diabetes; anticoagulants, which prevent blood from clotting; lithium, a drug used to treat various psychological problems; and diuretics, or water pills. In other words, *always inform your doctor of all medications you are taking.*

Can I take aspirin with my anti-inflammatory drug?

Aspirin and the anti-inflammatory drugs listed above result in similar side effects, especially gastrointestinal problems. Therefore, when they are taken together, the chances of a complication are increased.

In other words, don't mix aspirin with the anti-inflammatory drugs. The same holds true for over-the-counter ibuprofen, which like aspirin is an anti-inflammatory drug in high doses.

What do you do if you get the flu or have a fever? It is usually safe to mix acetaminophen with anti-inflammatory drugs, but of course don't do so without the consent of your physician.

I am allergic to aspirin. Is it OK to take an anti-inflammatory drug?

As discussed previously, aspirin allergies are manifested in two major ways — asthma and a skin reaction called urticaria. *If you are allergic to aspirin, or to any other anti-inflammatory drug, you are potentially allergic to all anti-inflammatory drugs.* Be sure to tell your doctor about all your drug allergies!

There may be an exception to the above. A group of aspirin derivatives called non-acetylated salicylates are often well tolerated by patients allergic to aspirin. Discuss this with your doctor.

I'm having surgery. Is it OK to continue my anti-inflammatory medication?

Since anti-inflammatory medications compromise the blood's ability to clot, *be sure to tell the surgeon what medications you are on* — even if it is aspirin or over-the-counter ibuprofen.

As previously mentioned, aspirin must be stopped ten to fourteen days prior to surgery. The other anti-inflammatory drugs should be stopped approximately five days prior to surgery. What can you take in the meantime? Usually acetaminophen. Although it does not have anti-inflammatory properties, it will reduce pain without reducing your blood's ability to clot.

I find it difficult to take drugs. Do I have to take anti-inflammatory drugs regularly?

The goal of therapy is to reduce inflammation

to the greatest extent possible. In order to accomplish this, anti-inflammatory drugs should be taken regularly. The object of therapy is to prevent inflammation, not reduce it once it occurs.

With all the anti-inflammatory drugs available, it is easier than ever to find one that is convenient and well tolerated. The medications that are taken once or twice a day may be most convenient for you. If you have trouble with pills, there are liquid forms available, as listed at the end of the chapter.

Patient compliance — or the ability to conform to a specific schedule of taking medications — improves with drugs that are taken once or twice a day, compared with medications taken three or four times a day. The convenience of the less frequent schedules is magnified in patients taking other medications in addition to their anti-inflammatory drugs.

Never alter your dose schedule by yourself, even if you think you're feeling better. Always consult your doctor.

What happens if you're one of those people who have trouble tolerating anti-inflammatory drugs? Modern medicine has at least some of the answers.

Is there anything I can do to decrease the

risk of developing gastrointestinal problems?

Although most people tolerate anti-inflammatory drugs when appropriate precautions are taken, some simply cannot. In addition, some patients have a prior history of ulcers. Are there any safeguards for these individuals?

First and foremost, routine safety measures must be taken. These include the precautions listed above such as taking the medication after a meal and avoiding excessive alcohol. Should these measures fail, there are a number of medications that often prove invaluable.

Antacids

One of the simplest approaches is to take the medication with an antacid. One hint: liquid antacids are generally more effective than antacid pills.

If you have gastrointestinal symptoms associated with anti-inflammatory medicine, you may feel the urge to put this book down, go to the corner pharmacy, and purchase a bottle of antacids. What you should really do is call your doctor, who should always be informed of the development of side effects. Some physicians will ask you to stop your arthritis drug (which is what I usually do), treat the gastrointestinal problems, and reintroduce an anti-inflammatory drug at a later date.

Misoprostol (Cytotec®)

One of the major advances in the treatment of arthritis patients in the last few years has been the development of a drug, misoprostol, that specifically prevents stomach ulcers caused by anti-inflammatory drugs. The explanation for misoprostol's success is as follows.

Anti-inflammatory drugs exert numerous chemical effects on the body, one of which is to decrease the production of a group of substances called prostaglandins. Prostaglandins cause inflammation, but they also have positive effects such as protecting the lining of the stomach. Unfortunately, no anti-inflammatory drug is smart enough to say, "I'll get rid of those bad prostaglandins in the joints but leave the good prostaglandins in the stomach alone." The result is a decreased level of prostaglandins in both places, which is good for the joints but bad for the stomach. Misoprostol is a prostaglandin; that is, to some extent it replaces the prostaglandins lost by action of the anti-inflammatory drug. Of course, not everyone on anti-inflammatory drugs develops ulcers, but for high-risk patients, misoprostol appears to be quite helpful.

Misoprostol may be associated with specific side effects, including diarrhea and abdominal cramping. These problems usually occur relatively early in therapy, frequently within the first few days, and then often disappear.

A more serious complication sounds a bit strange — misoprostol may precipitate labor in a pregnant woman. The explanation for this is quite logical. The same prostaglandins that cause inflammation and protect the stomach also induce uterine contractions. In fact, prostaglandins are used to induce labor. So the prostaglandin you take to help your stomach may also precipitate labor. *If you are a woman of child-bearing age, discuss these issues with your physician. Never begin therapy unless you are absolutely sure you are not pregnant. You must use effective contraceptive measures while on this medication.*

At the present time, misoprostol is the only drug approved by the Food and Drug Administration to prevent stomach ulcers caused by anti-inflammatory medication. It has not been shown to prevent duodenal ulcers and is not used to treat ulcers or prevent other symptoms associated with the use of anti-inflammatory medication.

There are a number of other drugs used to protect the stomach from the gastrointestinal effects of anti-inflammatory medications, as listed below. These drugs are not specifically approved by the FDA for the prevention of stomach ulcers. They are often used to treat gastrointestinal symptoms that arise in conjunction with anti-inflammatory therapy. Your doctor may administer them to you if you have a prior history of gastrointestinal problems, have developed problems while taking anti-inflammatory medication in the past, or have a prior history of a duodenal ulcer. *Don't forget to tell your doctor about your past medical history. It may influence your present treatment.*

Sucralfate (Carafate®)

This drug is thought to exert its action by protectively coating the stomach and duodenum. It is relatively safe, its major side effect being constipation, though it may also result in diarrhea. Other side effects include indigestion, dryness of the mouth, and dizziness.

Sucralfate may affect the absorption of a number of drugs, the most significant of which are tetracycline, which is an antibiotic; digoxin, which is used to treat heart conditions; and Tagamet®, which is discussed below. The solution to this problem is to separate the administration of these agents and Carafate® by at least two hours. The usual dose is one tablet four times per day on an empty stomach.

One hint: sucralfate is a rather large pill, and some people have difficulty swallowing it. You can get around this by dissolving it in a small amount of water and drinking the liquid.

H2 Antagonists

This is the term for a group of drugs that reduce the production of acid in the stomach. Acid is vitally important in the development of duodenal ulcers, less so with gastric ulcers. The drugs in this category include cimetidine (Tagamet®), ranitidine (Zantac®), and famotidine (Pepcid®). The choice of which agent to use and how and when to use it is quite individualized and varies significantly from physician to physician.

My doctor wants to put me on cortisone, but I've heard it's a dangerous drug. Should I take it?

If your arthritis is inadequately controlled by anti-inflammatory drugs, cortisone may be considered. Cortisone is a *corticosteroid,* or *steroid* for short. These substances are manufactured by the adrenal gland and are essential for a number of regulatory functions involving carbohydrates, proteins, and fats. They have significant anti-inflammatory effects. Synthetic cortisone compounds are used to decrease inflammation in a number of diseases, including various types of arthritis.

Corticosteroids have a number of potential side effects, and the decision to use them is a difficult one. Since they are such powerful drugs, they sometimes represent the only way severe bouts of arthritis can be controlled. They are given either in addition to anti-inflammatory drugs or by themselves and are administered orally, less frequently by injection into a muscle or intravenously, and by injection directly into a joint. Oral and intramuscular steroids are seldom used to treat osteoarthritis, but joint injections are sometimes used. Tendinitis, bursitis, and carpal tunnel syndrome are sometimes treated with direct steroid injections as well.

Steroid injections into joints are sometimes dramatically successful; on other occasions they are of little or no help. Most physicians are reluctant to do them on a routine basis; they are best reserved for treating acute flares. Infections are a very rare complication. Repeated injections may reduce the ability of cartilage to heal. Another fear is that joint damage may be accelerated if the joint is overused while the pain is being masked. Very little cortisone is absorbed into the body when a joint is injected.

Long-term steroid therapy, which is usually administered orally, is associated with a number of potential short- and long-term problems, which you should discuss with your physician. They include stomach upsets and the possible development of ulcers; increased appetite; fluid retention, especially in the upper body and face; increased blood pressure; acne; abnormal hair growth; thinning and easy bruising of the skin; increased blood sugar levels, or the temporary development of diabetes; osteoporosis, or thinning of the bones; muscle weakness; decreased blood flow to various joints, especially to the hip and knee, termed *aseptic necrosis,* which may cause major damage; menstrual irregularities; and emotional disturbances. Steroids may also precipitate episodes of glaucoma and cause cataracts.

It is apparent that steroids are potentially dangerous drugs. On the other hand, they are the most powerful of all anti-inflammatory medications and usually have a markedly beneficial effect. In fact, some patients feel so well on these medications that they don't want to decrease the dose or discontinue them. Steroids are used very reluctantly on a chronic basis, and your doctor will always use the lowest possible dose and try to get you off them as soon as possible. Their main uses are to treat acute flares that can't be managed by other means and as a "holding action" until a remission-inducing agent, as described below, has an opportunity to work.

When you receive steroids for more than a few weeks, your own adrenal gland stops making them. Doses are decreased slowly in order to give the adrenal gland time to increase production. A complete return to normal may not occur until you have been off steroids for one year.

Steroids should never be abruptly stopped. This may not only make your arthritis flare but make you very ill besides. Always be sure you have an adequate supply of this drug on hand.

Stress increases the body's need for corticosteroids. If you have been off the medication for less than one year and are exposed to a stressful situation, such as surgery or a serious infection, it may be necessary to supplement your body's supply of cortisone with a synthetic product. Therefore always include the fact that you've received cortisone in the past as part of your medical history.

My doctor wanted to inject a steroid into

my knee, but I was concerned because it is such a dangerous drug. Was my concern justified?

As noted above, steroids are indeed potentially dangerous, but injecting them into a joint is not the same as taking them orally and need not arouse the same apprehension. The long-term problems cited above do not occur after an injection, although a small amount of the steroid is indeed absorbed into the body. I have frequently heard patients with rheumatoid arthritis say they generally felt better after a cortisone injection into a single joint. This is no doubt because of the generalized absorption of the drug but is a short-lived phenomenon.

Severely swollen joints are often quite painful. Discomfort is often reduced, at least temporarily, by removal of joint fluid even if steroids are not injected. The fluid often reaccumulates; this may be reduced by the steroids.

Anti-inflammatory drugs don't control my arthritis. Can anything else be done?

There is an entire category of drugs that can be used should anti-inflammatory drugs prove inadequate. They are most often used to treat rheumatoid arthritis and are referred to as *disease-modifying* or *remission-inducing* agents. As the names imply, these medications are capable of putting the arthritis into remission. Unfortunately, they are not universally successful. They often produce only a partial improvement and sometimes do not work at all. Since these medications may take weeks or months to work, anti-inflammatory drugs are continued while waiting for a response to occur. If complete control occurs, the anti-inflammatory drug may be eliminated; more often it is kept at the same dose or reduced. When remission-inducing drugs are discontinued, disease activity almost always returns. Since these medications have been associated with severe side effects, their use is reserved for cases of severe, progressive disease.

A brief description of the drugs in this category follows.

Hydroxychloroquine (Plaquenil®) and Chloroquine (Aralen®)

These drugs are termed antimalarials because they are used to treat malaria. It was discovered quite by accident that they are useful in treating rheumatoid arthritis as well. They are given orally and may take weeks or months to work. These compounds may be deposited in the eye and result in a variety of visual problems. Decreased color vision and a decreased field of vision are the most common complications, but they occur rarely. Since an eye doctor can detect problems before they are noted by the person taking the drug, it is mandatory to see an eye doctor periodically — usually every three to six months. Other side effects include skin rashes, nausea, and diarrhea.

Gold Compounds

Gold is used to treat both rheumatoid and psoriatic arthritis. It is administered orally in the form of *auranofin* (Ridaura®) and by injection into muscle in the form of *gold sodium thiomalate* (Myochrysine®) and *aurothioglucose* (Solganal®). The oral form is taken daily. The injectable form is given weekly, and, if there is improvement, injections are reduced to every two, three, or four weeks. It may take up to four to six months for these preparations to work. If improvement does not occur by that time the medication is stopped.

Both types of preparations are associated with a number of potential problems, including rashes, sores in the mouth, and kidney and blood complications. Auranofin causes more gastrointestinal problems, such as loose stool or abdominal pain, than the injectable medications but is generally safer and is stopped less frequently because of side effects. These drugs are sufficiently dangerous that patients must be followed closely by the physician. Laboratory tests are diligently monitored — in the case of the injectable forms they are usually obtained prior to each injection.

Penicillamine (Cuprimine®, Depen®)

This drug must be discontinued in thirty to sixty percent of patients because of the development of side effects. These include skin rashes, nausea, and diarrhea. An unusual side effect is a decrease or loss of taste perception. Blood and kidney problems are potentially serious. If you are on this medication, your doctor will obtain frequent blood and urine tests. This is one of the few medications used to treat arthritis that is best taken on an empty stomach — at least one hour before meals or two hours after meals. It may take a number of months for this drug to work. If the initial dose is unsuccessful, the dose is very gradually increased. Depen® comes in 250-mg scored tablets, so it can be cut in half. Cuprimine® is available in 125-mg and 250-mg capsules. Some patients prefer the capsules, some the tablets.

Sulfasalazine (Azulfidine®)

This medication is used to treat rheumatoid arthritis and may be beneficial in ankylosing spondylitis. It is also used to treat ulcerative colitis. The most common side effects include rashes, headaches, and gastrointestinal symptoms such as decreased appetite, nausea, vomiting, and indigestion. The drug may also result in a decreased sperm count, which rebounds once the medication is withdrawn. Blood abnormalities occur rarely but may be serious.

Immunosuppressive Agents

These drugs have a direct effect on the immune system and are occasionally used to treat severe, progressive cases of rheumatoid arthritis. They are often used to treat other serious diseases such as cancer and may be associated with a number of potentially serious side effects, which your doctor should discuss with you in detail. The most frequently used immunosuppressive agents are as follows.

• Azathioprine (Imuran®) — Generally speaking, the dose used to treat arthritis is less than the dose used to treat cancer and is therefore usually safer. Complications include nausea; decreased white blood cell, platelet, and/or red blood cell levels; and liver inflammation.

• Methotrexate (Rheumatrex®) — This medication is usually administered weekly, either in a single or multiple doses. Complications include decreased white blood cell and/or platelet counts; ulcerations in the mouth; nausea, vomiting, and diarrhea; rashes and hair loss; and lung and liver abnormalities. Liver abnormalities are reduced by eliminating alcohol.

Is gout treated differently from other types of arthritis?

The treatment of gout can be very complicated. Anti-inflammatory medications are used to treat acute attacks. In selected patients, a drug called *colchicine* is used to treat as well as prevent attacks. In other patients, medications such as *allopurinol* (Zyloprim®), *probenecid* (Benemid®), or *sulfinpyrazone* (Anturane®) are utilized to rid the body of uric acid and so eliminate further attacks of gout, usually within six months to a year of beginning treatment. Colchicine is often taken to prevent attacks during this interim period.

Uric-acid-lowering medications must be

taken continuously or the uric acid will build up again. Not everyone with gout requires these medications. Whether or not you take them depends on your physician's judgment as well as your commitment to taking daily medication on a lifelong basis. Allopurinol decreases the rate at which the body produces uric acid in the blood, while probenecid and sulfinpyrazone increase the ability of the kidney to remove it from the body. Since probenecid and sulfinpyrazone increase the amount of uric acid in the urine, they may lead to the formation of kidney stones. The chances of this happening are reduced by drinking large amounts of fluid, which keeps the urine dilute. You should not be given these medications if you have had uric acid kidney stones in the past. You should also not take aspirin if you have gout; it may cause an attack, and it also blocks the effects of pro-benecid and sulfinpyrazone.

Discuss these issues with your doctor. There is no reason to suffer from gout.

Is there any way of treating Reynaud's phenomenon?

The cornerstone of therapy for this disease, in which the hands and feet become excessively cold (see Chapter 5), is to keep as warm as possible by wearing multiple layers of clothing, mittens, a hat, and so on. It is almost impossible to treat in the face of continued tobacco use.

Although the FDA has not approved a medication to treat this condition, many doctors use a variety of drugs that are also used to treat high blood pressure and heart disease. These are called calcium channel blockers. They appear to be promising drugs in the treatment of Reynaud's phenomenon. Discuss them with your physician if you are bothered by cold weather.

Is there any way to treat osteoporosis?

The emphasis here should be on prevention. An adequate amount of calcium and vitamin D in your diet, as well as regular exercise, are essential (see Chapter 10). If you are at high risk to develop osteoporosis, discuss bone density testing with your doctor (see Chapter 7) to detect the condition as soon as possible. Estrogens appear to retard the development of osteoporosis. If you can't take estrogens, calcitonin (Calcimar®), a synthetic hormone that prevents the loss of calcium from bone, may prove beneficial. It is injected under the skin, like insulin, usually on a daily basis. A number of experimental drugs are also being evaluated to treat osteoporosis.

A lightweight plastic shield that is worn over the hips is currently being tested. It may decrease your chances of fracturing a hip if you fall.

Osteoporosis is no longer a condition to be ignored. Discuss the pros and cons of therapy with your doctor.

Now, new uses for old drugs.

In addition to anti-inflammatory drugs, my doctor suggested I take an antidepressant to treat my arthritis. I'm not depressed. What good will it do?

Antidepressants are being used more and more to treat patients with chronic pain, no matter what the cause. It isn't clear how they decrease pain, but they seem to be especially effective in people who are having difficulty sleeping. They have proven reasonably successful in treating fibromyalgia and back pain but are also being used to treat many different types of arthritis. Some patients with arthritis are depressed about their condition and benefit psychologically from the use of these medications. The doses of antidepressants used to treat pain are often less than those used to treat depression, so the potential side effects are less as well. Since these can differ from medication to medication, be sure to discuss them with your doctor.

A final word about medication. As you can see, the choice of which medication to use and when to use it is a complicated one. A good medication for one person may be dangerous for another. Therefore, *never lend your medications to others and never use someone else's drugs — no matter how safe you think they are.*

Generic Name	Brand Name	Pill Sizes	Average Daily Dose Range
diclofenac	Voltaren ®	25, 50, 75 mg	100-200 mg in 2, 3, or 4 doses
diflunisal	Dolobid ®	250, 500 mg	500-1000 mg in 2 doses
fenoprofen	Nalfon ®	200, 300, 600 mg	900-2400 mg in 3 or 4 doses
flurbiprofen	Ansaid ®	50, 100 mg	200-300 mg in 2, 3, or 4 doses
ibuprofen	Motrin ® Rufen ®	300, 400, 600, 800 mg; liquid suspension	1200-3200 mg in 3 or 4 doses
indomethacin	Indocin ®	25, 50 mg; 75 mg slow-release capsule; liquid suspension; suppositories	75-200 mg in 3 or 4 doses
ketoprofen	Orudis ®	25, 50, 75 mg	150-300 mg in 3 or 4 doses
meclofenamate	Meclomen ®	50, 100 mg	200-400 mg in 3 or 4 doses
naproxen	Naprosyn ®	250, 375, 500 mg; liquid suspension	500-1000 mg in 2 doses
phenylbutazone	Butazolidin ®	100 mg	variable; seldom used for more than one week
piroxicam	Feldene ®	10, 20 mg	20 mg in one dose
sulindac	Clinoril ®	150, 200 mg	300-400 mg in 2 doses
tolmetin	Tolectin ®	200, 400, 600 mg	600-1800 mg in 3 doses

9

Other Forms of Treatment

In addition to medication, there are many ways to treat arthritis. This chapter describes a number of conventional approaches that are offered by physicians and allied health professionals, including nurses, physical therapists, occupational therapists, social workers, and dieticians. These approaches are often neglected by physicians, especially those who do not specialize in the field of arthritis.

When placed on medication, many patients ask, "Will I have to be on this forever?" One way of improving your chances of eliminating medication is by taking advantage of the types of treatments discussed in this and subsequent chapters.

What takes place in the offices of allied health professionals simply represents the beginning of your treatment. For example, physical therapists teach you exercises, but you must do them at home. Occupational therapists make suggestions regarding changing your environment, but you have to institute those changes.

In other words, it's up to you.

Besides taking medication, what else can I do for my arthritis?

As mentioned previously, the treatment of arthritis is a multi-pronged affair. Among your physician's first goals are to control your discomfort and maintain normal joint motion and muscle tone. To accomplish this you may be sent for *physical therapy*.

The goal of physical therapy is to relieve pain and maintain or restore use of the involved joints and their surrounding muscles and tendons. A number of methods are employed, including exercise and the application of heat and cold, as described below.

On occasion, you may be sent for physical therapy without being placed on an anti-inflammatory medication; that is, your physician may feel that physical therapy alone will suffice. This is only true for minor problems and is virtually never the case for rheumatoid arthritis. Your doctor may also send you to physical therapy for treatment of tendinitis or bursitis.

Another allied health care provider, the *occupational therapist*, also has an important role. Occupational therapists concentrate on the hands and provide exercises and various types of therapy designed to reduce discomfort and maintain normal function. In addition they determine the work capabilities of their patients, both inside and outside the home, and make suggestions for modifying the home and work environment in order to make their patients' lives more functional and less stressful.

Your physician may also suggest you see a *dietician* if you need help with your diet. Many patients with osteoarthritis have a tendency to be overweight, and this may have a deleterious effect on the joints as well as on overall health. More specific information regarding diets appears in the next two chapters.

Finally, you may be depressed and not function well emotionally because of your arthritis. This sets up a vicious cycle. The worse you feel, the more depressed you get; depression then makes your arthritis feel even worse. It's essential to break this cycle. A specially trained nurse or social worker can prove invaluable in this regard.

Thus the treatment of arthritis is an all-encompassing affair, and often includes individuals besides your physician.

What do physical and occupational therapists do specifically?

Since there is an overlap between what physical and occupational therapists do, they will be considered as one. Physical and occupational therapy come under the heading of *rehabilitation medicine,* the aim of which is to maintain or restore function. Physical and occupational therapists use a number of tools and approaches, referred to as *modalities of therapy,* as described below. Some may be used as part of a home treatment program as well as in the therapist's office.

Heat

The application of heat is one of our oldest ways of treating pain. Heat makes joints and muscles more comfortable and loosens them up prior to range-of-motion and stretching exercises. In fact, other than an improved sense of well-being, the most important purpose of heat is to relieve pain and reduce muscle spasm sufficiently to allow each joint to go through a full range of motion and to permit muscle-strengthening exercises.

There are two main types of heat, superficial and deep. The most common way of delivering *superficial heat* is by simply taking a shower or bath, which should be warm but not hot. Many patients with arthritis routinely do this upon arising and before exercise.

Superficial heat is most easily delivered by hot compresses or dry or moist hot packs, which are also called hydrocollators. Most patients find moist hot packs to be more effective. Superficial heat is also delivered by whirlpool and by wax or paraffin baths which are discussed below.

Here are a few hints for using heat.

- The heat should be mild and make you feel comfortable, not hot.
- Optimal time for heat application is 15 to 20 minutes. It should rarely if ever be applied for longer periods.
- Do not lie on the heat source — it should be placed on top of the area being treated.
- Place a protective layer, such as a cloth or towel, between your body and any kind of heat pack.
- If you use a topical preparation for pain relief that contains a menthol gel, remove it before applying heat. Otherwise it can lead to a severe burn.

An unusual way of administering heat to the hands or feet is by applying a coating of wax. This is initially applied in the therapist's office, but if successful, home kits are available. The patient repeatedly dips the hands or feet into a wax bath, and the wax hardens quickly, sealing in the heat. The involved areas are then wrapped in plastic bags and warm towels for approximately 15 to 20 minutes. Since the wax is premixed with mineral oil, it then peels off rather easily. Patients often find this quite helpful but frequently object to the home program, which can be laborious.

The most common way of delivering *deep heat,* or *diathermy,* is by a system called *ultrasound.* Ultrasound reaches joints more effectively than superficial heat. It is also a valuable aid for treating tendinitis, bursitis, and deep muscle spasm.

Heat is most often used in the treatment of chronic conditions. It should not be applied to swollen or severely inflamed areas or areas with poor blood supply or impaired sensation.

Cold

Application of cold results in decreased pain and swelling. It is used for both acute and chronic arthritis and for acute sprains and strains.

Some patients find it very useful to apply cold to a chronically involved joint or tendon immediately after engaging in exercise; for example, to an arthritic knee after walking or to a shoulder plagued by chronic tendinitis immediately after playing tennis.

Here are a few suggestions regarding cold.

- An inexpensive way of providing cold treatments is by filling a plastic bag with crushed ice. You can also purchase reusable gel-filled cold packs.
- Protect your skin with a thin cloth or towel — don't place the cold pack directly on your body.
- Optimal time for application is approximately 10 to 15 minutes. Don't apply cold packs for more than 20 minutes.
- Don't apply cold packs if you have poor circulation.

Heat and/or Cold

The application of heat or cold is less than a scientific proposition — if one doesn't work, the other often will. In fact, many people utilize both; for example, heat before exercising, cold applied directly to the involved joint immediately after exercising, then a warm shower. Others use alternating heat and cold for pain relief. A commonly used method is two to three minutes of heat followed by a minute of cold. The process is then repeated two or three times.

Often used together with the application of heat, massage is primarily designed to decrease muscle stiffness and spasm. It increases blood flow and warms the involved area. It may also decrease pain. Although the manner in which this is accomplished is unclear, the stimulus provided by the massage seems to compete with that generated by the source of pain, and the brain senses the former. Even when massage does not reduce pain, it is often quite relaxing. Some patients find it reduces their stress level, at least temporarily.

I prefer that massage be administered by a physical therapist or other health care professional, as opposed to a massage therapist who may not be familiar with specific medical problems. If you find massage helpful, learn to do it yourself. Muscles in the arms, legs, and neck are most accessible. Using powder or baby oil sometimes makes it easier to work on your muscles. Some find that application of a topical menthol gel results in additional pain relief. A few warnings regarding self-massage: stop if it results in pain, don't massage an inflamed area, and be careful not to hurt other involved joints, such as the wrists, when administering massage.

A technique called *friction massage* is used

to treat tendinitis. This involves deep pressure applied over the tendons, usually by the thumbs. It probably breaks up scar tissue and helps restore circulation to the inflamed tendon.

Electrotherapy

A device called a *transcutaneous electrical nerve stimulator,* or *TENS unit,* can often decrease arthritis pain. This consists of a battery unit and electrodes, which are attached to sites of pain. The electrodes are turned on and off as needed. The theory behind this is that pain can be blocked by "over-stimulating" the surrounding nerves. Relief may begin promptly, often within minutes, and may last for hours or days. Unfortunately, everyone does not respond to this form of therapy, but for those who do it may be extremely helpful.

Patients who are pregnant or have heart problems or pacemakers should avoid electrotherapy.

Traction

Traction is applied by a series of weights and pulleys or by a machine. It is an accepted form of therapy to improve decreased range of motion in joints such as the wrist, elbow, hip, and knee. Its use in the treatment of spinal problems is more controversial. Theoretically, one would think that traction applied to the spine would pull apart diseased vertebral bodies, allowing more normal alignment and therefore taking pressure off "pinched" nerves. The problem is that over two hundred pounds of traction applied for thirty minutes is necessary to pull apart vertebral bodies in the low back, or lumbar spine, yet pelvic traction only consists of twenty-five to fifty pounds, so it is unlikely to work in that fashion. Since it does seem to work for some people, it may do so by stretching tight muscles. A more skeptical explanation is that the bed rest associated with traction is most responsible for any improvement that may occur.

Traction for the neck, or cervical spine, is used more often, but some still question its efficacy. Although cervical traction probably also works by stretching tight muscles, only thirty pounds of traction is necessary to increase the space between individual cervical vertebral bodies. Since typical cervical traction is between fifteen and twenty-five pounds, this at least approximates the theoretical pressure required to pull apart the diseased joint spaces.

Traction should always be used cautiously

and only by experienced people. In general, orders for traction are written by physicians and the procedure administered by physical therapists.

Splints

One of the most effective ways of reducing inflammation is by resting a joint, and one of the easiest ways of accomplishing this is by the use of a splint. Wrist and finger splints are commonly used, and they are usually custom fabricated by the occupational therapist. Patients are often self-conscious about using these devices, so they may only be used at night, and this is frequently sufficient to markedly decrease inflammation and make the joint more comfortable. Should pain persist, they are also used periodically during the day, especially when performing stressful tasks.

The suggestion that splints be worn at night deserves some comment. After all, aren't we resting at night anyway? We actually move around quite a bit when we sleep, although this decreases as we grow older. The use of splints at night allows the splinted joint to rest totally so that optimal healing can occur. This improvement carries over into the next day.

A number of other devices accomplish the

same thing as splints; that is, they rest the involved areas. These include neck collars, back corsets and braces, and knee braces. Special devices to help the feet are also available. Canes and crutches are used to help reduce stress on joints such as hips and knees. They can be surprisingly effective. For example, a cane can reduce the weight on a joint by as much as fifty percent. Incidentally, the cane should be held on the side opposite that with the most symptoms.

These devices should always be carefully fitted, and you should be instructed in their use.

Although the rest of my arthritis is better, my feet just aren't improving. Any suggestions?

Under these circumstances your doctor may ask you to see a podiatrist. *Podiatry* is the branch of medicine that specializes in the foot. Podiatrists study at schools of podiatry, not medical schools, and receive the degree of Doctor of Podiatric Medicine (D.P.M.).

It is often very difficult to treat arthritis in the feet using only anti-inflammatory drugs. Because we must walk on our feet all day long, we continuously traumatize them, so the inflammation gets no chance to heal.

Podiatrists are ingenious when it comes to devising various support systems, such as pads and bandages, that take the stress off inflamed joints.

Some people have naturally poor foot posture. Examples of this are flat feet, high rigid arches that don't "give" and therefore poorly absorb the body's stresses, and ankles that always seem to be caving in or out. These problems may lead to local arthritis or tendinitis. If you have a generalized condition such as rheumatoid arthritis that also happens to affect your feet, these conditions can make the arthritis even worse. Under these circumstances the podiatrist may elect to fashion an *orthotic*, a form-fitting mold you wear inside your shoe or sneaker. Because it is individualized, it can be built up where your foot needs extra support. The result is that your foot anatomy is made as normal as possible, your joints and tendons are less stressed, and you feel better.

Structural problems in the foot can lead to problems in other areas of the body. If the foot cannot adequately absorb stress, the stress may be transmitted to the knees, hips, or back. This is especially true if there are pre-existing conditions in any of these areas.

I am reminded of a 27-year-old woman, Betty Allison, who consulted me because of back pain. An avid runner, she was especially frustrated because running clearly worsened her back problems. She had seen her family doctor, who thought she was suffering from back strain and appropriately sent her to physical therapy, where she was taught various back exercises. These, along with rest, virtually eliminated the back pain. But every time she tried to run the pain would return.

One of the first things I did was examine her feet. She was incredulous, but I reasoned that since her back was being appropriately treated, at least part of the problem might be coming from elsewhere. Indeed, she had a number of foot problems, and I sent her to a podiatrist who fashioned a pair of orthotics. Within a few weeks she was back to running and was virtually pain-free.

Betty did have a minor problem in her back, but it was worsened because her feet could not properly absorb stress. This meant that the stress was ultimately transmitted to her back, making a mild problem significantly worse. After she started wearing the orthotics she still had to do her back exercises, but the combination of the two resulted in a major improvement.

What kind of exercises should I do if I have arthritis? Can the therapist help me with them?

There are two categories of exercise — therapeutic and recreational. Therapeutic exercises are prescribed by your doctor or therapist with specific goals in mind. Recreational exercises are discussed in the next chapter.

The goal of therapeutic exercise is to preserve or restore normal range of motion in the involved joints and to maintain or increase the strength of the muscles surrounding each joint. These are termed range-of-motion and muscle-strengthening exercises, respectively, and represent the two major types of therapeutic exercise.

A joint's *range of motion* represents all the movements of which it is normally capable. Patients with arthritis should move their joints through their full range of motion on a daily basis. This is accomplished by range-of-motion exercises, which not only prevent loss of motion and deformities but also reduce stiffness and pain.

Many patients do not completely understand the value and importance of these exercises. They do not understand that *normal daily activities do not put joints through their full range of motion*. For example, extend your arms straight over your head. This motion is seldom used during the normal course of the day. Even reaching to put something on a high shelf rarely produces this extreme motion. Yet it is important to move your joints fully in order to preserve their function. Also, if a joint is painful we are less likely to move it, and ultimately motion will be lost.

Similarly, daily activities are seldom adequate to strengthen muscles — hence the need for specific muscle-strengthening exercises. Muscles originally weaken when they are not fully used by painful arthritic joints. Once weakness develops, it can worsen the arthritis. Impact is normally absorbed to a great extent by muscles. Once they weaken, their ability to perform this function decreases, and more and more impact is transmitted to the joints. This extra stress in turn worsens the arthritis.

There are two kinds of strengthening exercises. *Isometric exercises* tighten muscles without moving joints. They are ideal for patients with arthritis because they allow muscles to be strengthened while only minimally stressing joints. The other type of exercise utilizes light weights or some other form of resistance. These put more stress on the joints and should only be initiated by a therapist.

Your physician or therapist may suggest a water exercise program. There are a number of advantages to exercising in water. It is buoyant, resulting in less stress on the joints, but it also offers some resistance. Most people also find the water comfortable and soothing.

Exercise programs are individualized according to the severity and extent of a person's arthritis. On some occasions the patient may simply be taught a set of exercises by the therapist. The patient then does these at home, usually every day. At the other end of the spectrum is a program in which the therapist actively helps the patient move the joints or provides resistance in order to strengthen the involved muscles. These programs usually require that the patient go to physical therapy two to three times a week, although daily home exercise is also required. These programs are also likely to involve the various treatment modalities discussed above.

Incidentally, once you reach the point where you can exercise independently at home, the time commitment is relatively brief, usually about ten to fifteen minutes a day.

What can I do to ensure maximum benefit and safety from an exercise program?

There are a few rules you should follow to make your exercise program as safe and beneficial as possible. The following apply to a therapeutic exercise program, be it in the therapist's office or your home, as well as to a recreational program.

- Do therapeutic exercises daily. This maximizes joint improvement. More vigorous conditioning and recreational exercises should be done three to four times a week.
- Exercise when you are feeling relatively well during the course of the day. For example, if you have severe morning stiffness, it may be worthwhile to do some simple stretching exercises after an early shower but to leave more vigorous exercises, including strengthening and recreational exercises, for later in the day. The important thing about exercises is that you do them, so schedule them when they are most comfortable and convenient.
- Take advantage of the modalities of therapy discussed above, such as heat and cold, before and after exercise programs as needed. Your doctor and therapist will discuss what is best for you, and from that point it is a matter of trial and error until you find the right individual formula.
- Do more strenuous exercise approximately two hours after a meal. Avoid exercising on a full stomach.
- Start your exercise program slowly, and build it up gradually. Don't be discouraged. You may not have exercised in a long time, and it may take quite a while before you even begin to approximate

your goals. But you will get there.

- Always warm up before vigorous exercises and cool down afterward by decreasing the pace of the exercise while your breathing and heart rate gradually return to normal. Never stop exercising abruptly. It is often useful to do your stretching exercises before and after a more vigorous program. For example, if you are accustomed to doing stretching exercises every morning, do these even if you plan additional exercise, such as a game of tennis, later in the day. However, repeat the stretching exercises before and after the tennis.
- Wear clothing that is warm, loose, and comfortable. Wear comfortable shoes with nonskid bottoms. The shoes should also give you good support.
- Avoid getting chilled, as this may increase muscle tension. If need be, wear an extra layer of light clothing, which can be discarded as you warm up.
- Stop the exercise if it results in significantly increased pain, especially if it is more pain than you are used to. A bit of increased discomfort may be acceptable — this varies according to your condition, so discuss it with your physician and therapist. However, *increased pain should*

not last for more than one to two hours after the exercise has been completed and should not result in increased pain or stiffness the following morning. If any of the preceding occur, simply do less the next time until you find a comfortable level. Do not abandon the exercise program unless the pain is severe or does not go away. Under these circumstances, discuss the situation with your physician. Once you begin to improve, your exercise tolerance will improve as well, and you will ultimately be able to expand your program.

- Never "force" a joint to move.
- If your joint is inflamed, move it very gently through its range of motion. Inform your physical therapist of changes in your condition so your exercise program can be modified accordingly. For example, you may require active assistance while doing some of your exercises.
- Never use weights when a joint is actively inflamed or if use of the weights results in pain.
- Move your joints slowly and smoothly, giving your muscles time to rest between repetitions. Avoid jerking motions.
- Learn to breathe properly while exercising. Don't hold your breath while going

through range-of-motion or strengthening exercises. Exhale when doing the active part of your exercise. For example, if you're doing a sit-up, inhale first, then slowly exhale as you're doing the sit-up.

- Avoid exercising to the point of fatiguing your joints and muscles. Usually you can maintain normal muscle tone and preserve range of motion by doing less than ten repetitions. However, you will have to find out what is right for you.

- Since the activity of your arthritis may vary, your exercise program may vary as well. Do more when you're feeling well, less when you're not, but still do therapeutic exercises daily. Don't set specific exercise goals that must be met on a weekly basis — you may be setting yourself up for disappointment. Also, some people do less when they're feeling better, as decreased pain often translates into decreased motivation. "I didn't think I had to exercise, because I was feeling so much better" is a typical explanation. But patients may feel better *because* they have been exercising, and by not doing so they may be depriving themselves of a major component of their therapy. In addition, it is important to get in as good shape as possible in preparation for a time when you may not be able to exercise as actively as you would like. Once you are doing your prescribed exercises, you should be able to begin a general exercise program as well. More on this in the next chapter.

- Stop exercising if you develop a muscle cramp or pain. Rest, then gently massage the involved area. It is usually appropriate to continue the exercise once you feel better, but exercise more gently.
- Finally, if you develop shortness of breath, tightness across your chest, chest pain, dizziness, or feel sick to your stomach or faint, *stop exercising immediately*, lie down, and inform those around you of your condition.

The therapy made me feel worse. Should I stop?

Going to physical therapy represents a commitment of time and effort. Usually I ask my patients to see the therapist two to three times a week for at least a month and often longer. It is not unusual for patients to feel a bit worse at first, but the difference should be minor and short-lived. In other words, a bit of increased discomfort while the therapist is working on you is permissible, but this should be mild and disappear within an hour. It should not carry over into the evening or the following morning. If it does, the therapist may not be doing the right thing or may be too aggressive. The solution to this problem is not to abandon therapy — it is to tell the therapist what is happening so the treatment can be modified.

Are there any practical things I can do to reduce arthritis pain in everyday life?

Therapists will teach you how to protect your joints from stress while doing everyday tasks. This is called *joint protection*. Overuse of joints may result in increased inflammation, as manifested by increased pain and swelling, and ultimately lead to increased joint damage and loss of function. Some principles of joint protection follow.

• Pay attention to pain. Don't persist in tasks that increase discomfort — there are usually ways to modify your activities. As noted in the exercise guidelines above, you should not experience pain that lasts for more than one to two hours after completing a task or that results in significantly increased pain and stiffness the following morning. Should either of these occur, modify your approach to the activity — do it differently or take more breaks.

• Staying in one position often leads to increased stiffness and pain. Change positions frequently or take breaks as often as necessary. Discover what works for you. If you're writing a long letter or working at a typewriter or word processor for a prolonged period of time, relax and stretch your fingers, wrists, and arms every five to ten minutes — or more or less, depending on your individual condition. In general, you shouldn't sit for more than an hour without getting up and stretching.

• Avoid or modify activities that result in sustained stress to joints; for example, tasks that necessitate a tight grip.

• Use the palm, not the fingers, for pushing or turning. Opening a screw-top jar ordinarily requires a sustained tight finger grip. Instead, lean on the jar lid with your palm and turn it by using a shoulder motion. This assumes, of course, that your shoulders are doing relatively well compared with your fingers. Similarly, spread your palm over a sponge rather than gripping it with your fingers.

• Avoid twisting motions and sudden forceful motions needed to overcome an object's inertia, such as turning a tight door knob or lifting a heavy object.

• As a corollary to the above, slide rather than lift heavy objects.

• If you must lift, do so by bending at the knees, keeping the back straight. (This has to be modified if you have knee problems.)

• Use both hands and arms to lift, and keep the object as close to your body as possible. Don't abruptly jerk the object, but lift it gradually and smoothly.

• Always use good posture. It puts less stress on your joints and muscles. For example:

— *Sitting*. Use a firm chair with armrests. This reduces pressure on your shoulders and back. Your knees should be slightly higher than your hips. Keep your feet flat on the floor. Your back should be straight.
— *Standing*. Distribute your weight evenly on both feet. Relax your knees. If standing for a long time, place one foot on a footstool to decrease back tension.
— *Sleeping*. Use a firm mattress. If you lie on your side, keep your knees bent. Don't put pillows under your knees.

• Always use the largest or strongest available joint.

— When lifting or carrying, distribute the weight from your fingers and wrists to your forearms and shoulders. Don't shift the weight to a more severely involved joint.

— Carry a purse by a shoulder strap as opposed to a hand grip.

— Open doors with your body, not your hands.

— When going up stairs, lead with your stronger leg. When going down stairs, lead with your weaker leg.

— Everyday maneuvers such as getting out of a chair can be simplified by using the correct technique. Keep your feet flat on the floor, tucked in as close to the chair as possible. Obtain leverage by placing your palms on either the arms or the seat, lean forward, and push up with your hips and knees. Specially designed seats situated higher off the ground than usual make this easier as well.

• If possible, work in a seated rather than a standing position. This can be quite important to someone doing assembly line or clerical work. Don't be afraid to talk to your employer about modifying your job.

This last point was dramatically illustrated to me by Edna Davis, a 56-year-old woman who did assembly line work at a company

211

that manufactured small electrical components. She consulted her internist because of right hip pain. He made the diagnosis of osteoarthritis and placed her on an anti-inflammatory drug. When she did not improve he suggested she see me. She said her hip almost never bothered her on weekends, just during the week and toward the end of the day. She explained the nature of her job, and I didn't give it a second thought. She kept insisting her job was to blame, but I didn't understand, having wrongfully assumed she sat down on the assembly line. When I finally realized differently, I asked her to speak with her employer and request that she be allowed to sit. Her employer responded positively, and her work situation was changed. The result was an almost complete disappearance of her hip pain. Edna's osteoarthritis was so mild that it required a whole day of standing before she developed her symptoms.

This is a perfect example of what can be accomplished by a rather simple change in the workplace to protect an arthritic joint.

Speaking of modifying the workplace brings us to the next question.

Are there any ways I can change my surroundings to make my arthritis feel better?

The therapist will analyze how you function at home and in the workplace and offer suggestions designed to improve both. This is called *analysis of activities of daily living*. Some of these suggestions will entail principles of joint protection, as described above. In other cases specific devices will be recommended to simplify your daily routine.

Examples of how to make routine activities easier by special devices and adaptation of the environment follow.

Personal Hygiene and Dressing

• Many patients with arthritis find it difficult to rise from toilets, which for the most part are built quite low. A raised toilet seat helps solve this problem. Guard rails improve the safety of the toilet and can also be used around the bath. Always remember to put a safety mat in the bathtub. It is sometimes helpful to sit on a plastic seat in the shower. Keep towels within easy reach to reduce the need for bending and stretching.

• There are many aids to facilitate dressing and undressing. These include long-handled shoe horns and button and zipper hooks. Add small chains to zippers to facilitate grasping. It may prove worthwhile to replace buttons with Velcro if buttoning and unbuttoning give you a lot of trouble. Consider the use of slip-on shoes or shoes with Velcro closures. Be sure these are well fitted, as they often do not give the support of tie shoes. If you have trouble tying ties, a pretied one may be the answer. Finally, do as much of your dressing in a sitting position as possible.

• Long-handled brushes and toothbrushes make personal grooming easier. An electric toothbrush often proves particularly helpful. These devices also have thick handles, which makes gripping easier. There is a dental floss holder that can be held in one hand, eliminating the need for a number of two-handed manipulations within your mouth. Pump dispensers for toothpaste are easier on the fingers than squeezing a tube.

Food Preparation and Eating

• Consider using a high stool when cooking or working at the counter or sink. The kitchen should be designed to minimize reaching and bending. Keep frequently used appliances such as toasters on the counter, not in a cabinet. Similarly, keep pots by the stove. As many shelves as possible should be at counter level, and cabinets should have pull-out shelves. If you have high shelves, place only light objects on them and use a long-handled reacher to get them down. Shelves should be relatively shallow in order to minimize reaching. These same principles apply to any workplace.

• Use lightweight pans, such as those made out of aluminum. Try to find one with compartments so you can cook more than one thing in the same pan. Build up pan handles to make them easier to grip.

• Take advantage of modern technology by using food processors, electric knives, electric can openers, blenders, and dishwashers. However, some people find washing dishes by hand relaxing, the exercise beneficial, and the warm water soothing.

• Many simple devices are available that make it easier to open jars. An old-fashioned pair of pliers with soft grip handles can be used for a number of kitchen tasks, such as opening milk cartons, removing wraparound seals from frozen juice cans, and opening tab cans. In fact, it's sometimes easier to open the latter by using an electric can opener and forgetting about the tab.

• When baking, line pans with aluminum

foil, and use nonstick products or Teflon pans when frying. This reduces cleanup time and effort.

• Plan your menu as far in advance as possible and shop accordingly. This minimizes last-minute, inconvenient trips to the store. Also, consider cooking a little extra so the additional food can be used in the future in lieu of a completely new meal.

• There are a number of adaptive devices, such as utensils with built-up handles, to make eating easier. Use mugs with large handles instead of cups with small ones. Use insulated glasses to hold your iced drinks to protect your hands from the cold.

The Home

• Allow others to share the responsibility. For example, if you do the washing and drying, sort each family member's clothes into a separate basket and allow *them* to put them away. Try to plan ahead so you don't have to do more than one major cleaning job a day, or do the easiest and ask another family member to do the others.

• Whenever possible, perform household

chores like ironing, sorting, and folding clothes while sitting. Store cleaning materials and implements where they are to be used rather than in a central place. For example, if you have two bathrooms, keep cleaning detergents and brushes in both of them. If you have a two-story house, consider keeping a vacuum cleaner on each floor. A self-propelled vacuum is easier to manage than one where you have to supply all the pushing energy. An electric broom, which is less expensive, could substitute on one floor if appropriate. While on the subject of keeping things in the same place, use an apron with pockets so you don't have to make extra trips to retrieve cleaning materials.

• Use a feather duster with a long handle to reduce reaching and bending.

• An automatic toilet bowl cleaner reduces the number of times the bowl must be scrubbed. When cleaning the toilet or bathtub, use a long-handled mop.

• Consider putting casters on furniture that is frequently moved. Have a high-seated chair in each room — they're easier to get in and out of. Be sure upholstered furniture such as couches is not too soft — you may sink so low it may be difficult to stand.

• There are a number of adaptive devices that can be placed over doorknobs to facilitate turning.

• For lawn and gardening work, use light-weight tools with long handles to reduce reaching and bending. When kneeling use a soft pad to protect your knees. Consider a snowblower or mower you can ride on if you want to continue to do heavier outdoor work.

The Workplace

• An adjustable swivel chair with good back support is a necessity. The height of the chair should be adjusted so your arms rest comfortably on either the work surface or the arm rests when your feet are flat on the floor.

• When writing at a desk or table or when using a computer terminal, try to sit as upright as possible while bending your neck only slightly. This produces the least amount of stress. If you find this difficult, put your feet on a footstool. This virtually forces you into the correct position and is quite comfortable. Another alternative is to use a drafting table with an adjustable slant. This reduces neck and upper back strain.

• Organize your desk or work area so that frequently used items are close by. Use stacking trays to increase the number of objects within easy reach.

• Felt tip pens require less pressure than ballpoints. Use thick-handled pencils or use an adapter, the original intent of which was to make grasping pencils easier for children. It is available in most stationery stores. Similarly, use thick-handled tools.

• A simple book holder can significantly reduce strain on the hands, wrists, and arms.

• Take advantage of modern technology by using power tools and electric staplers and pencil sharpeners. Dictating equipment reduces the amount of writing you must do, but avoid small hand-held units with miniature controls. Consider sending tape recordings to friends in lieu of letters.

• Word processors are generally preferable to electric typewriters, which in turn are preferable to manual typewriters.

• A push-button phone is easier to use than

a dial phone. If you use the phone frequently, a speaker phone will reduce stress on your hand, wrist, and arm.

The Automobile

• Power steering and brakes, power window controls, cruise control, and heated seats are luxuries that make being in your automobile a lot easier. Similarly, power seat controls allow frequent changes in position while driving. This can benefit the entire body — obviously the back, but also the hips, knees, shoulders, elbows, wrists, and hands. Try a back support if you develop back discomfort while in the car. An overhead strap makes entering and exiting easier.

• A car door opener and an ignition adaptive device simplify these tasks. Use an antifreeze spray in the winter to make it easier to turn door locks.

• An automatic garage door opener eliminates the need for lifting the garage door and also keeps you in your heated car during the cold winter months.

• If you are thinking of going from a standard shift to an automatic transmission, be sure to check the locking mechanism on the gearshift. Some of these require intense thumb pressure to operate. Also, when considering a new car, remember that bucket seats may look good but are often hard to get out of.

• Test drive a new car extensively before making a purchase. Be sure you are comfortable in it. Don't assume you will get used to minor problems.

This is far from an exhaustive list. If you're having trouble with a task, no matter how simple it is, tell the therapist, or, if you haven't seen one, request a consultation. There are usually ways to solve your problems.

Even if you apply all the above principles in your home life, other problems may occur. This is illustrated in the next question.

My husband gets upset when I can't keep up with my household tasks. I keep trying harder, but there is only so much I can do because of my pain. My marriage is starting to suffer. Any suggestions?

Just as the family can be a wonderful support for the patient with arthritis, it can also be a source of anguish. The divorce rate among people with arthritis is significantly higher than in the general population, and part of the problem may be partners' differing perceptions. A recent study done by researchers at the University of North Carolina examined work perceptions of married couples. Women with arthritis and their spouses often differed markedly in their assessment of the woman's ability to do household tasks. The men both over- and underestimated their wives' disability. It is important that the person with arthritis and the spouse understand the severity of the disease because a misunderstanding can add enormous stress to the marriage.

So be open about communicating with your spouse, but be aware that even that may not be enough. Spouses have their own psychological ways of dealing with their mates' problems, and it may be necessary to involve a physician or counselor to be sure both partners in the relationship are looking at the situation realistically.

Application of some of the approaches discussed thus far can effectively treat one of the arthritis sufferer's most common laments.

My morning stiffness is sometimes so bad I have a hard time getting to work on time. My doctor changed my medicine a few times,

but it hasn't helped enough. Any suggestions?

There are practical things you can do to reduce morning stiffness and pain. Since joints may stiffen in the cold, be sure to keep warm while you are asleep. An electric blanket may prove useful in this regard. Purchase a timer that can be linked to your thermostat so the heat goes up before you get out of bed. Do some stretching exercises upon arising, or immediately step into a warm shower and do them there.

If you like getting up to a hot cup of coffee, connect a timer to an electric coffee pot. By the time you get to the kitchen your first cup will already be ready! Lay out your breakfast foods and utensils the night before to reduce preparation time the next morning. Also lay out your clothes the night before — it can make getting going in the morning a lot easier.

The treatment of arthritis is admittedly a complicated process that takes a lot of hard work on the part of doctor and patient alike. What happens if things don't go as well as we would like? The following question is usually asked at that time.

I'm doing so poorly — why don't you just put me in the hospital?

This question is actually much more complicated than it sounds and must be answered on a number of different levels.

From a medical perspective, hospitalization certainly has its benefits. Medications arrive on time. Meals are nutritious if not overwhelmingly appetizing — and someone else has the responsibility of cooking them. You are removed from your work environment, whether it is inside or outside the home. This usually results in decreased stress, which, as outlined in the next chapter, is exceedingly important. In addition, assuming the hospital has an active rehabilitation medicine department, physical and occupational therapists are available on a regular basis. Social workers may be of value if you are experiencing emotional problems or adjustment difficulties. It is sometimes worthwhile to have a family conference with the various health care providers so they can better understand your medical and psychological problems.

The downside of hospitalization is that insurance companies are reluctant to pay for care, such as physical and occupational therapy, that can be rendered on an outpatient basis. By using all available resources, it is often possible to avoid hospitalization. The visiting nurses' association can check your condition and see that medications are taken.

Physical therapy at home can be arranged. A home aide can help with personal hygiene and household chores as well as food preparation. Arrangements can be made for meals to be delivered to the home.

Of course you are still surrounded by the stresses of your home environment. In addition, it is often difficult to feel comfortable with and depend on an endless flow of strangers coming to your home.

Fortunately, patients with arthritis rarely require either hospitalization or an aggressive home program as detailed above. But if you're not doing well, don't hesitate to ask for help. Be totally honest with your physician — it's the only way to get the help you need.

What's the role of surgery?

When medication, physical and occupational therapy, proper nutrition, and other forms of conservative therapy prove inadequate, surgery may be considered. But the mere thought of surgery is often so frightening that its role must be put into perspective. Most people with arthritis will never require surgery. However, for those who do, the benefits are often quite impressive. The main reason for surgery is usually pain relief. Surgery may also produce an increased ability to use your joints, and it may correct deformities, which may result in cosmetic improvement, especially when the hands are involved. The most frequently performed surgical procedures are as follows.

Synovectomy

This refers to the surgical removal of the *synovium*, or lining of the joint. Radioactive isotopes injected into the joint may achieve similar results — this experimental procedure is currently being evaluated. Normally paperthin in width, the synovium becomes inflamed and proliferates madly in rheumatoid arthritis. It can mushroom from a tissue barely discernable under the microscope to one easily seen by the human eye. In fact, overgrown synovial tissue may be noted by patient and doctor alike, especially in the fingers and wrists, elbows, and knees. The various chemicals capable of destroying bone and cartilage originate in the synovium.

Synovectomy is considered when a joint fails to respond to standard medical therapy. Although synovectomy may successfully reduce pain and swelling, the synovial tissue may regrow.

Although synovectomies are done for a host of joints, including the shoulders, elbows, hips, and knees, one specific type of synovectomy deserves specific mention. Patients with rheumatoid arthritis are prone to develop a condition termed *dorsal tenosynovitis* (*dorsal* means "back," *teno* means "tendon," and *synovitis* means "inflammation of the synovium"), which involves the tendons on the back of the hand. The tendons are attacked by the proliferating synovial tissue, become inflamed, and sometimes tear or rupture, causing loss of movement in the finger to which the involved tendon is attached. A synovectomy may be done in anticipation of a tear or to prevent additional tendon tears after one has occurred. The torn tendon may be repaired at the time of surgery as well.

Arthroscopy

This innovative procedure enables the surgeon to look into the joint with a thin lighted tube called an arthroscope. Direct visualization of the joint can be an invaluable diagnostic aid, and the surgeon can often determine the type and extent of the arthritis as well as the presence of other problems such as a torn meniscus (see Chapter 7). The latter can often be repaired, as minor surgery can be performed through the arthroscope. More extensive surgery, such as a synovectomy, can occasionally be performed as well. The major advantage of arthroscopic surgery is that the joint is not surgically opened, so recovery and rehabilitation occur relatively quickly. Less anesthesia is usually required as well. Surgeons will often do arthroscopic surgery to determine the nature and extent of a problem, and if it is too involved to be repaired through the arthroscope, proceed with a more traditional operation. Arthroscopic surgery is most often done on the knee and shoulder, but someone skilled in the art will do other joints, such as the elbow and ankle, as well.

If arthroscopic surgery had been available in 1968, the course of Bobby Orr's career might have been dramatically changed. Injuries such as his are now routinely repaired through the arthroscope, allowing relatively prompt return to the activities of daily life and even to the rigors of playing a professional sport.

Arthrodesis

This means the fusing together of bones. In essence it eliminates the involved joint, thus removing the source of discomfort. It is most often done in the thumb, wrist, and ankle. The diseased area is strengthened by the procedure but flexibility is lost.

Resection

The removal of part or all of a damaged bone is called a resection. It is indicated when affected bones in the feet make walking painful and is frequently quite successful. This type of procedure is also utilized to remove bunions, which may be painful, unsightly, and make it difficult to find a properly fitted shoe.

Osteotomy

The goal of this surgical procedure is to restore normal anatomy to an arthritic joint. It is accomplished by cutting or remodeling bone so that weight winds up being more evenly distributed. It is often considered an alternative to total joint replacement (see below), especially in an individual under the age of 50.

Total Joint Arthroplasty

Here the joint is removed and replaced by an artificial one. This can eliminate relentless pain emanating from a hopelessly destroyed joint and restore a significant measure of function to a joint long rendered useless.

As I tell my patients, total joint replacement is analogous to dental extraction of an abscessed tooth. Once it's out, there's no more pain. In fact, some patients notice pain relief as soon as they awaken in the recovery room. However, just as the dentist prefers to save your diseased tooth and thus maintain the normal anatomy of your mouth, the surgeon first does everything possible to restore and preserve the integrity of the joint with procedures such as synovectomy and osteotomy, as described above. The timing of these operations is of critical importance, as they should not be done before medical therapy has had an opportunity to work but should be performed before extensive joint damage has occurred. These principles are particularly applicable to the young, active individual since "the real thing" is preferable to an artificial joint — it feels better and functions better. Another reason for delaying total joint replacement is that artificial joints may not last indefinitely.

For the most part artificial joints have been cemented in place, and this has proven to be the weak link in the procedure. Loosening of the joint is a potential problem, especially in young patients whose activity hastens the failure of the cement. Nevertheless, most total hip replacements have lasted more than ten years.

Cementless joint replacement is a new procedure that may solve the problem of cement failure. The implants used in this type of surgery are porous, allowing bone to grow into the artificial joint, thus forming a more stable union. Since cementless joint replacement is a relatively new procedure, it remains to be seen whether it will prove better than cemented joints. However, many surgeons consider it very promising, especially for young patients and in situations where the original surgery failed and another operation is deemed necessary.

Total hip and knee replacements are commonly performed operations done with a high degree of success. Artificial shoulders and elbows are implanted less frequently, and total wrist and ankle replacements are experimental. Finger joint arthroplasty is also available. Although often successful in reducing pain and improving the appearance of the fingers, it is less successful in restoring motion than arthroplasties involving other joints.

How can I prepare for surgery?

If you are contemplating joint replacement, or any type of joint surgery for that matter, you must take a number of things into consideration. These include the following.

• Choose your doctor and hospital carefully. Find a surgeon you are comfortable with who has specific expertise in joint surgery. More on this in Chapter 15.

• It is often advisable to get a second and even a third opinion. If you are seeing a rheumatologist who suggests a particular type of operation, and you then see a surgeon who agrees, it is probably unnecessary to get another surgical opinion, although some insurance carriers may require it.

• Since most joint surgery is elective and does not have to be done immediately, prepare for the surgery by getting yourself in as good shape as possible. Have your primary care physician perform a routine exam to identify any hidden problems that might have a negative impact on the surgery. This is a great opportunity to lose weight if indicated. Weight reduction makes both the operative and post-operative courses easier. Excess weight puts extra stress on your heart and lungs during surgery and on your joints, especially weight-bearing joints such as the hip and knee, afterward. Excess weight will also interfere with your rehabilitation exercises.

• Your doctor will probably discuss the

issue of *autotransfusion* or *autologous transfusion* with you. This entails donating your own blood in the weeks prior to the operation so that you can receive it during or after surgery as needed. The safest blood you can receive is your own.

• Be sure to review your medications with your primary care physician and surgeon because you may have to alter them prior to the operation.

• Surgery is only the first step in rehabilitating a joint. Postoperative physical therapy is vital, perhaps as important as the original surgery! Do your exercises as directed. If you were in a lot of pain prior to the surgery, there's a good chance muscle weakness developed around the involved joint. This will make your physical therapy harder, but don't get discouraged.

• Pay attention to your doctor's orders regarding rest, activities, medication, and so on. Don't cheat — you're only cheating yourself.

• Be sure your family members are involved in planning the operation and understand their responsibilities thereafter. This may result in some alterations in their usual routines, but it will only be temporary.

• Have realistic expectations or you will be setting yourself up for disappointment. Your new joint will never be as good as your original joint, and you must accept that. But it will be a lot better than your arthritic joint.

Still undecided about the virtues of joint surgery? Consider the following.

After I finished my medical training I took a cross-country camping trip. In the Southwest I visited a national park that offered a rather strenuous guided tour of ancient Indian ruins. It took approximately half an hour to reach the ruins. The trail was narrow, a bit windy, and mostly downhill. Most of the people on the tour were under the age of 40, but one couple appeared to be in their 70s. As it turned out, my estimates were right. On the way back I struck up a conversation with the man, who was 73. His wife was 71. I told him how impressed I was with both of them for going on the tour. He smiled and said the person I should really be impressed with was his wife. Three years ago she had been confined to a wheelchair with arthritis in both hips. Reluctant to have surgery but desperate to escape from her wheelchair, she finally consented to undergo two total hip replacements. Now she was keeping up with people less than half her age.

It's a wonderful story and shows what can be accomplished if you don't give up hope. Surgery may not be for everyone, but it's a Godsend for some.

10

Taking Control — Ways to Help Yourself

The spirit of self-help is the root of all genuine growth in the individual . . . Help from without is often enfeebling in its effects, but help from within invariably invigorates.

          — SAMUEL SMILES (1812 – 1904)

One of the most common questions the patient with arthritis asks is, "Can I do anything to help myself?" In the past the physician often answered with a woeful shrug and advised taking medication, perhaps doing a few simple exercises, but little else.

How times have changed! The responsibility for treating arthritis is now shared by physician and patient. Now more than ever we appreciate the importance of "simple things" such as diet, rest, exercise, and stress reduction. Adherence to sound health care principles is vitally important to the person with arthritis. Disregarding those principles has an even more deleterious effect on the arthritis sufferer than on the normal individual.

Racquetball champion Lynn Adams speaks eloquently about the principles of self-care. "As an athlete you try to control everything in your environment so you are in control, not your opponent, not the crowd, not the referee. The more you do that the greater the likelihood you'll succeed," she says, and she applies the same ideas to her arthritis. "What can I do so I can gain control over the disease? I can't believe there's not always something." In both aspects of her life she does anything she can do "to have an edge." For example, by incorporating the principles of joint protection discussed in the previous chapter, she has learned to shift stress from a painful to a comfortable joint. She knows the value of rest and changes her schedule to accommodate her needs. She watches her diet and does not smoke or drink. As a result, only three matches in her career have been affected by her arthritis.

Actress Alice Faye is another strong believer in the importance of self-care. A major motion picture star during the thirties and forties, she appeared in over forty motion pictures, including such hits as *On the Avenue* in 1937 with Dick Powell, *Alexander's Ragtime Band* in 1938 with Tyrone Power and Don Ameche,

Rose of Washington Square in 1939 with Tyrone Power and Al Jolson, and *Lillian Russell* in 1940 with Don Ameche, Henry Fonda, and Edward Arnold. Born in 1915, she is afflicted by osteoarthritis of the hands, back, and toes. For the last seven years she has toured the country as a representative of a major pharmaceutical company delivering health care information to other "young elders." She has received a number of awards for her work in this field.

Alice Faye urges her audiences to "stay active and involved," exercise regularly, eat a well-balanced diet, avoid tobacco, and see their physicians regularly. And she practices what she preaches, eating wisely and either walking or swimming daily.

Juliet Prowse, introduced earlier in this book, is another arthritis sufferer who has taken control of her disease. She understands the importance of taking the medication as prescribed by her physician. She adheres to a vigorous exercise schedule yet knows the importance of rest. A gourmet cook, her diet is healthy and sound. A devout believer in the importance of a sound mind in a sound body, she practices yoga to reduce stress. Hobbies such as needlepoint serve as a form of relaxation. In short, she does everything possible to help herself.

Just as Lynn Adams, Alice Faye, and Juliet Prowse have taken control of their disease, so can you.

The most often voiced questions about self-help follow.

Do patients with arthritis require a special diet?

We have already established that we have no irrefutable scientific evidence to suggest that anything in the diet either causes or cures arthritis (see Chapter 3). However, that doesn't mean diet isn't extremely important to the patient with arthritis. Whether you are suffering from a generalized form of joint disease such as rheumatoid arthritis or a local problem such as osteoarthritis of the back or knee, adherence to sound dietary principles can be extremely helpful.

First of all, the diet should be well balanced, with all the major food groups appropriately represented. The goal should be maintenance of normal body weight. This sounds as if it shouldn't be a problem, yet a study published in 1963 indicated that the typical patient with rheumatoid arthritis is ten pounds underweight. Various investigators theorize that this relative malnutrition may contribute to the inflammatory process and does not fully allow healing to take place. Extreme examples of this are concentration camp and famine victims. Both groups suffer from a number of medical problems, one of which is difficulty in wound-healing.

The same study indicated that patients with osteoarthritis average fifteen pounds above their recommended weight. The added weight certainly has a negative effect on the joints, especially weight-bearing joints such as the hips and knees. This is true no matter what type of arthritis you have. Some researchers believe that excess weight is actually one of the causes of osteoarthritis, especially of the knees, and especially when the individual is extremely overweight.

A number of factors influence the nutritional status of the patient with arthritis. Pain and fatigue may decrease one's appetite. Patients with arthritis who are depressed about their condition may have a decreased appetite, but they may also overeat as a way of dealing with their emotions. When this occurs, the wrong foods, such as ice cream, cakes, and cookies, are often consumed. Finally, there may be practical problems regarding food preparation.

Older patients with arthritis, and some younger ones as well, may also suffer from heart disease or high blood pressure. Weight control is vitally important to these conditions.

Since achieving a well-balanced diet is often easier said than done, you should consider taking a multivitamin to help ensure good nutrition. Proper nutrition contributes to the normal function of the immune system, but vitamins taken in excess may prove dangerous. Therefore, consult your physician or a dietician before proceeding along these lines.

Similarly, supplementary minerals, such as calcium, may prove helpful. Individuals with arthritis are often less active than their peers. Inactivity accelerates the development of osteoporosis (see Chapter 7). This may be at least partially prevented by the addition of calcium and vitamins. The latter are required because vitamin D is responsible for the normal absorption of calcium. At a minimum, your diet should contain the National Research Council's Recommended Dietary Allowance (RDA) of calcium, which is 1000 mg per day for adults. Postmenopausal women are at greatest risk to develop osteoporosis and require 1200 to 1500 mg of calcium per day because the ability to absorb calcium from our diets decreases as we grow older. Increased calcium supplementation for men is less important because they do not develop osteoporosis as frequently as women.

The most recent (10th edition) of RDAs increased the amount of calcium suggested for individuals between the ages of 11 and 24 to 1200 mg per day. The rationale behind this is to make the bones as dense as possible while an individual is still developing so that later in life, when bone loss occurs, there will be more of a built-in reserve.

Most people in our country do not get enough calcium in their diet. This is especially true of women of childbearing age, who incidentally often don't get enough iron either. Unfortunately, many of the foods that are rich in calcium also have a high fat content. A few important exceptions are listed in the following table.

Food	Calcium (mg)	Calories
cheddar cheese (1 oz)	204	115
mozzarella/part skim milk cheese (1 oz)	183	72
skim milk (1 cup)	302	85
yogurt (1 cup)	415	145
yogurt with fruit (1 cup)	345	230
fish (3 oz)		
salmon	167	120
Atlantic sardines, canned in oil, drained, with bones	324	175

Green vegetables, especially broccoli, are relatively good sources of calcium as well.

Using the above as a guide, in order for young adults to obtain adequate calcium from their diet they have to drink four glasses of milk, preferably skim or low fat, or eat three cups of yogurt per day.

If you can't get enough calcium in your diet, discuss with your doctor the possibility of taking calcium supplements. A warning — don't go overboard. Excess calcium can cause kidney stones. Also, be sure to remind your physician if you've had kidney stones in the past.

Finally, steroids can cause osteoporosis, so if you're on this medication be sure to ask your doctor about the value of calcium and vitamins and perhaps other medications to combat this effect.

You should also emphasize protein and carbohydrates in your diet. Fats should be reduced in order to keep cholesterol as low as possible. There is little doubt that cholesterol is a major risk factor in the development of heart disease. Increased risk is associated with a cholesterol value of 240 or above. Values between 200 and 240 are considered border-line, and values below 200 are considered optimal. However, the situation is confusing because there is more than one type of cholesterol. Low-density lipoproteins (LDLs), the so-called "bad cholesterol," accumulate in arteries and cause heart disease. High-density lipoproteins (HDLs) are "good cholesterol" because they decrease LDLs.

Why is this particularly important to the arthritis sufferer? Because HDL level is influenced by exercise to some degree. The more you exercise, the greater the chance you will reach your optimal HDL level. Since people with arthritis often cannot exercise as much as they would like, there may be a tendency for the HDL level to go down. If they aren't exercising and not eating the right foods, the LDL level will go up. This is a bad combination. Low levels of HDL may also be hereditary. HDL level can be raised by losing weight and not smoking, as well as by exercise.

If your cholesterol is elevated, change your diet. The National Cholesterol Education Program of the National Heart, Lung, and Blood Institute recommends a diet with less than thirty percent of total calories from fat, less than ten percent from saturated fats, and less than 300 mg of cholesterol per day. The average American's present diet is thirty-seven percent fat.

Animal products rich in fat include whole milk, butter, cheese, and ice cream. Although beef is often incriminated, some beef is low in saturated fat. Vegetable fats high in saturated fats include cocoa butter, which is found in chocolate, coconut oil, palm kernel oil, and palm oil. These are found in factory-made baked goods, cake mixes, and nondairy substitutes, among others. You can lower your cholesterol by eating fewer egg yolks. Try not to eat more than three or four eggs a week. Try to substitute two egg whites for each whole egg in recipes.

The good news is you may be able to decrease your cholesterol by as much as ten to fifteen percent, and perhaps more. Levels of cholesterol and LDL often begin to drop within two to three weeks of going on an appropriate diet. This doesn't mean you have to give up food high in saturated fats forever. Once you've reached an optimal level, an occasional indulgence does not materially alter your cholesterol.

While on the subject of indulgences — fat contributes up to fifty-five percent of the calorie content of the typical fast-food meal, considerably more than the recommended thirty percent. Even fast-food chicken may contain a significant amount of fat because of the way it is prepared. In addition, some large fast-food sandwiches contain twice the daily recommended allowance of salt. Please, do not make a habit of eating fast foods!

A good policy for many is to place more emphasis on carbohydrates and decrease fats, even if your cholesterol is not significantly elevated. The body "burns off" carbohydrates but stores fats. It's easy to gain weight from excessive fats in the diet, and that has a potentially deleterious effect on the joints. Starchy foods are good sources of carbohydrates. These include breads and cereals, potatoes and corn, and rice and pasta.

So keep your fats down and your carbohydrates up. Even the active individual with an increased HDL level may benefit from reduction in cholesterol.

Don't forget to include fiber in your diet. Fiber-containing foods help avoid constipation, which can afflict anyone but is more likely to be a problem for the older patient with arthritis who is relatively inactive. Foods rich in fiber include fruits, vegetables, and whole grain breads and cereals.

People with arthritis should keep their diets as low in salt (sodium) as possible. This is especially true for people who are relatively inactive. Sodium leads to fluid retention, which can be worsened by inactivity. In addition, inactivity can lead to weight gain, which in turn can lead to increased blood pressure, which in turn is worsened by sodium. Some medications, such as corticosteroids, may result in sodium retention as well. If any of the above apply to you, your physician may recommend a specific low-sodium diet.

Those with rheumatoid arthritis are wise to restrict the amount of sugar in their diet. People with this type of arthritis often suffer from Sjogren's syndrome, an inflammation of the lacrimal and salivary glands (the glands that produce tears and saliva, respectively), as described in Chapter 5. The result is an initial decrease in the quality of tears and saliva, then a decrease in their quantity as well. Abnormalities of saliva lead to an increase in the number of cavities. If you have rheumatoid arthritis and suffer from dryness of the mouth, you probably have this complication. However, Sjogren's syndrome may be present even without this complaint. It is therefore advisable to avoid sugars.

This is a reasonable recommendation even if Sjogren's syndrome is not present, as sweets have few redeeming qualities. Admittedly, however, they taste good. It is unwise as well as unnecessary to deprive yourself totally. Remember, moderation in all things.

Finally, limit alcohol as much as possible. Alcohol consumption is often a contributing factor to weight gain because alcohol contains a large number of "empty" calories. In addition, alcohol can upset the stomach, as can anti-inflammatory drugs. The two simply don't mix very well. In addition, the regular use of alcohol appears to be associated with osteoporosis. Again, moderation is the key. Be sure to discuss your alcohol consumption with your doctor.

In summary, following a healthy diet makes *you* more healthy. It allows your immune system to work as effectively as possible, keeps your weight and blood pressure down, may allow you to live longer by decreasing your cholesterol, allows you to tolerate your medication better, and even preserves your teeth. You can't lose!

No matter what I do, I can't lose weight. Do you have any suggestions?

Keep a diary of everything you eat for three days — this will give you and your doctor a good idea where the problem is. Also note what time you eat your meals and snacks — and don't forget to put the snacks on the list!

Most Americans eat scanty breakfasts followed by a midmorning cup of coffee, perhaps with a doughnut. Then lunch, which is also usually light. By mid- to late afternoon the average person on the above diet is famished. A quick trip to a candy machine often follows, then a large dinner, and often a midevening snack. The latter often consists of fattening food such as cake or ice cream.

What's the solution? Eat a larger, healthy breakfast. If that doesn't have a "domino" effect on your eating habits for the rest of the day, eat a larger lunch as well. The object is to avoid end-of-the-day hunger, since that's the time most people crave sweets.

A few other hints. Get your fats from peanut butter — it's healthier than the fats in french fries and ice cream. Olive oil, peanut oil, and oils derived from vegetables are preferable to oil derived from animal fats and coconut and palm oils. As noted above, watch your alcohol intake. Salads are great but they often don't provide much in the way of nutrition. Remember, the darker the vegetable, the more nutrients it contains. Finally, watch out for the salad dressing — it may contain 400 or more calories. Some salads are simply a collection of foods low in nutritional value covered by a glop of calories!

Don't deprive yourself of everything you enjoy eating; that will almost certainly doom the diet to failure. Allow treats in moderation — especially after you've been particularly good for a period of time.

I advise my patients to weigh themselves once a week at the same time and under the same circumstances — for example, at ten o'clock Sunday morning, wearing the same robe. Since body weight often fluctuates on a day-to-day basis, it is unnecessary and can even be discouraging to weigh yourself more frequently. Over the course of a week everything will average out.

Successful weight loss is more analogous to running a marathon than a one hundred-yard dash. Weight that comes off slowly as a result of good eating habits is more likely to stay off than weight lost quickly. Aim to lose no more than one to two pounds a week.

That is by no means a complete treatise on how to lose weight, but it should get you thinking. By all means, bring that three-day list of your food intake to your doctor. If your doctor isn't interested, ask to see a dietician.

Finally, it is difficult to lose weight without an appropriate exercise program. Just because you have arthritis it doesn't mean you can't or shouldn't exercise.

I tend to avoid the range-of-motion exercises my physical therapist taught me because I find them boring. Any suggestions?

Many people find exercising boring. Here are a few suggestions that may help.

• *Schedule* your exercises. They are sufficiently important to be scheduled, not simply performed haphazardly. If you keep an appointment book or have a reminder calendar, write down when you are to exercise and be sure there are no conflicts.

In order to emphasize the importance of exercise I occasionally give patients prescriptions for exercise when it is apparent they are not working out regularly. The usual response is, "I don't need a prescription for this." I respond by saying that I want them to take their exercise as seriously as a prescription for medication. Most patients faithfully adhere to prescriptions for medication. They should view their exercises in the same fashion.

• Find ways to relieve boredom. For example, exercise to your favorite music or television show. Promise yourself that the only way you will watch a favorite show is if you do your range-of-motion exercises while doing so. Exercise in areas you find particularly pleasant, both inside and outside the home. Walking is a wonderful recreational or conditioning exercise. Try taking different routes around your home or driving to a park or your favorite part of town. Utilize the local school track.

- Another way of reducing boredom is to exercise with other people. This may prove to be socially as well as physically valuable.

- Keep a log that objectively measures your progress. You may not notice improvement on a day-to-day or week-to-week basis, but you will be surprised to see how much you accomplish in the long run. A log is a wonderful form of positive reinforcement. Logs monitored by your therapist or physician tend to work even better.

- If you are engaged in a regular conditioning program (as discussed below), have contingency plans should something interfere with it. For example, if you walk regularly, do you have any alternatives when the weather gets cold? One is to walk in a shopping mall, which has become an increasingly popular form of exercise. Another is to purchase an exercise tape that you can use at home.

- If you still can't stick to a regular program, discuss it with your doctor. It is a very important issue and should not be ignored.

Can I do recreational or conditioning exercises if I have arthritis? Are they a substitute for range-of-motion exercises?

This question raises important issues. Most people would obviously prefer tennis and golf to stretching or range-of-motion exercises. Recreational and aerobic or conditioning exercises such as walking and swimming are extremely important and *should be included as part of the overall treatment program if at all possible.* In fact, this is one area in which I believe I can be justifiably critical of my fellow physicians, including many rheumatologists: they simply do not adequately stress the importance of exercise.

The potential benefits of exercise are legion. Exercise helps us shed excess pounds and maintain a normal body weight. It preserves muscle tone, helps maintain normal range of motion of joints, keeps blood pressure down, increases cardiovascular fitness and thus reduces the risk of heart disease, and has an enormously beneficial psychological effect. Exercise is even good for your bones — in fact it is one of the cornerstones of the treatment of osteoporosis. Once patients with arthritis get into an active recreational or conditioning program, they frequently find that the added exercise makes their joints feel better. In short, exercise is one of the most important things you can do for yourself.

However, *recreational and conditioning exercises are a supplement to therapeutic exercises, not a replacement.* As noted in the prior chapter, therapeutic exercises are needed to maintain range of motion and muscle tone and decrease stiffness. Recreational exercises alone do not adequately accomplish this. So the person with arthritis ideally should do both types of exercises.

Every time I begin a more active exercise program my joints hurt. What do I do?

Most people with arthritis intuitively decrease their activities because of pain and so get out of shape. Now we want to reverse this process.

Once your physician has you on a regimen of medication and therapeutic exercise and your arthritis is under reasonable control, you are ready for a recreational exercise program. Don't proceed without your doctor's consent. Doctors may want to do additional tests (such as a cardiogram) to be sure you can tolerate your chosen program. They will also issue guidelines so you know how rapidly you can proceed; for example, how rapid your pulse rate should be.

You now add recreational exercise and find it increases your pain. What do you do?

The treatment of arthritis should not be designed simply to control the pain of an inactive individual; it should cover the relatively active person as well when at all possible. So tell your doctor and physical therapist if your increased activities result in increased discomfort. They may recommend, among other things, that you do your stretching exercises before and after recreational activities or that you be more aggressive regarding the use of heat and cold, as described in Chapter 9. In addition, your physician may suggest increasing the dose of your medication or perhaps changing it. If you begin slowly and increase your program gradually, you will probably ultimately note decreased discomfort. However, you still may be somewhat uncomfortable in the beginning.

I tell my patients that the aim of therapy is to allow them to lead as normal a life as possible, and I encourage them to do anything within reason to achieve that end. So don't be satisfied if you're comfortable at rest but in pain when you're active. You deserve more.

From a practical perspective, how do you begin your exercise program?

Choose an activity you *like* and start slowly. *Gradually* increase the time you spend exercising — the ultimate goal is four days per week for twenty to forty minutes per session. This is enough to strengthen your muscles, preserve your joint motion, and maintain cardiovascular fitness. Beyond that you increase the risk of injury but do not accrue an increased benefit.

An added benefit of moderate exercise is that it appears to keep people sexually fit well into their sixties. Too much exercise, on the other hand, can diminish sex drive.

Walking is an exercise that you can usually do safely on a daily basis if tolerated. If not, aim for every other day. Walking regularly is one of the healthiest things you can do for yourself and a wonderful habit to develop.

When I suggest walking as a form of exercise, many patients respond by saying they are on their feet all day anyway. It's not the same thing. In order to benefit from walking it must be done without interruption and in addition to your routine daily activities. Ideally it should also be done briskly enough to work up a sweat.

As with all exercises, begin gradually. Walk to the end of your block and back. Walk slowly. Assuming you have no ill effects, increase to one and a half blocks the following week. Try to increase the pace of your walk a bit. Before you know it, you'll be up to twenty to forty minutes.

If you can increase the pace of your walk, remember still to start slowly, gradually increasing the pace, and wind down slowly as well.

Maintain good posture while walking. This decreases the strain on your back and hips. Keep your head up, your shoulders back, and your chest out.

Harry Truman recognized the importance of walking and incorporated it into his daily schedule whenever possible. Another committed walker is *Life* magazine photographer Alfred Eisenstaedt. Born in 1898 in Prussia, he moved to New York City in 1935. Often called the father of photojournalism, he has taken some of the most memorable pictures of this century. Perhaps his most famous photograph is that of a sailor impulsively kissing a nurse in Times Square on V.J. Day. He has photographed the people who have shaped our contemporary world, including John F. Kennedy, Albert Einstein, Marilyn Monroe, and Sophia Loren, who remains a close personal friend to this day. As a tribute to his work he was awarded the National Medal of the Arts in 1989.

In his own words, Alfred Eisenstaedt has always been a "health bug." Intuiting the importance of exercise before it was popularized, he never wavered from his daily schedule of walking and calisthenics. Currently 91 years of age, his mobility has been decreased by osteoarthritis of the hips and knees, which has grown progressively worse over the last eight years. Disquieted by the thought of navigating the streets of New York City as a form of exercise, he walks around his apartment between twenty and forty times per day.

I spent a morning with Alfred Eisenstaedt in his office on the twenty-eighth floor of the Time Life Building in Manhattan where he still goes to work every day. It was clear that this is a man who just will not quit, who is going to keep moving until the day he dies. In fact, when I asked him when he was going to retire, he said, "I'll retire when I'm dead."

In addition to his arthritis, Eisie, as he is affectionately known, has had a heart attack, eye surgery, and trouble with his balance. Yet he still walks every day.

If he does it, so can you.

These men were ahead of their time in recognizing the importance of walking as a form of exercise. Now that this is common knowledge, there are no excuses.

If you prefer another exercise, swimming, biking (both stationary and outdoor), and low-impact aerobics are usually appropriate. The former is especially beneficial for the patient with arthritis.

Do the things you enjoyed in the past, such as golf and tennis. If singles tennis is too much of an effort, try doubles.

If you are discouraged, seek out an exercise class for patients with arthritis. Once an unheard-of venture, these classes are now readily available in many locations, and they can provide immeasurable peer support. Consult your doctor, the physical therapy department of your local hospital, or the nearest chapter of the Arthritis Foundation for further information.

Once you begin to exercise you will be amazed how much better your joints feel and how much better you feel in general. Don't get discouraged — it's a gradual process. The more you do, the more you'll be able to do.

Not convinced you can help yourself? Think of tennis star Jack Kramer, considered by many the greatest serve-and-volley player in the history of the game. His accomplishments are extraordinary: Wimbledon singles champion in 1947, Wimbledon doubles champion two years in a row, played on two winning Davis Cup teams, U.S. Professional champion five years in a row, member of the Tennis Hall of Fame, and the grandfather of what ultimately became open tennis, or professional tennis as we know it today. Kramer jokes that some people know him only as a piece of sporting goods equipment. The Wilson Jack Kramer wooden racket is the most popular

tennis racket in the history of the game —
10 million were produced from 1949 to 1981,
at which time metal replaced wood.

Jack Kramer is presently 69 years old, and
he has had arthritis since the age of 29 when
it first developed in his back and neck. His
initial reaction to the discomfort was typical.
Since rest and heat made him feel better, he
assumed he was suffering from muscle
sprains, a common problem among athletes.
But when the pain went to his shoulder and
affected his powerful serve, his whole game
suffered. He knew something was wrong, but
was nevertheless shocked when his physician
informed him he had arthritis. Rest, exercise,
and treatment with cortisone (a dangerous
drug, but its side effects weren't fully appreciated and there weren't many alternatives
— see Chapter 8) enabled him to continue
his professional career. In fact he won the
U.S. Championship that year, defeating
Pancho Segura — a testimony to his courage
and athletic ability. When he retired at the
age of 33 he was still the reigning U.S. Champion.

Ironically, he retired because of the effects
of the cortisone, not his arthritis. He realized
the drug was destroying his body, and it just
wasn't worth it. So in his own words, "I traded
in my racket for a business suit." He then

became one of the greatest promoters in the history of the game.

Unfortunately, without the anti-inflammatory effects of the cortisone his arthritis began to get the better of him. He became depressed as his tolerance for physical activity decreased. He gained weight and his cholesterol went up, as did his blood pressure. In short, his arthritis was not only threatening his lifestyle but his life.

But that competitive instinct wouldn't die. He kept seeking help. Arthritis had totally destroyed one of his hips, so he had a partial hip replacement. At least that made the hip pain go away, but he still couldn't do much.

His doctor finally found the right anti-inflammatory medication, and Jack took it from there. As soon as the pain subsided he embarked upon an exercise program to which he diligently adhered. He strengthened his muscles and joints. He dieted and lost the excess weight. His blood pressure came down, as did his cholesterol. He began to sleep better, and his disposition improved. Today Jack Kramer is once again an avid tennis player and golfer, participating in one or the other on an almost daily basis. He can beat men half his age in both sports. And he looks wonderful.

Still don't think anything can be done for arthritis? Ask this former Wimbledon champion. He's more active now than he was thirty years ago.

I've just started to exercise, and although I'm making progress I find it exhausting. Is there anything wrong with me?

It's normal to be fatigued after beginning an exercise program, especially if you've been inactive for a considerable period of time. As noted in the answer above, you get out of shape, or, as doctors call it, "deconditioned," if you don't exercise regularly. Just think how exhausted you are after emerging from a bout with the flu. After a few days of rest the average person is "weak as a kitten." Imagine the ravages of months, or even years, of inactivity. So don't be discouraged, but do mention the problem to your physician. There may be complicating factors contributing to the fatigue, but this is usually not the case. It took a long time to get out of shape; therefore it will take an equally long period of time to get in shape. But it can be done.

My joints hurt when I exercise, but I know how important exercise is and I don't want to give it up. Can I hurt my joints if I do too much? How do I know when to stop?

Although this issue has been touched on previously, it deserves emphasis. Unfortunately, you can injure your joints if you overdo physical activity. It's all right for your joints to hurt while you're exercising, but the pain should not be severe or unusual; it should not last more than two hours after you stop exercising or result in increased pain or stiffness the following morning.

If walking for fifteen minutes results in increased knee pain that lasts for two hours, you've done too much. The next time you walk, limit yourself to ten minutes. The resulting pain will probably be short-lived. If so, limit your walks to ten minutes for the next one to two weeks, and then try increasing to fifteen minutes. You'll probably tolerate the increase the second time around. Eventually, you'll find a regular exercise program that will leave you and your joints feeling better.

As a generalization, stay at each exercise level for one to two weeks before increasing your activities.

A former Wimbledon champ who has some rather strong opinions regarding the role of exercise in the treatment of arthritis is Vic Seixas. He won the Wimbledon singles championship in 1953 and the mixed doubles title from 1953 through 1956. He won the U.S. Championship in 1954 and played on seven

Davis Cup teams. In fact, he has played more Davis Cup matches than any other American, or fifty-five altogether. He was inducted into the Tennis Hall of Fame in 1971.

Unlike Jack Kramer, Seixas did not develop arthritis while still in his prime. However, he was still relatively young at 55, and actively competing in Grand Masters tournaments. It was at one such tournament that he first realized something was wrong.

"While playing in the Grand Masters, my knees started feeling achy and a little stiff," he recalls, "but I thought it would disappear with a little extra TLC. When it began getting worse instead of better, I went to my doctor and learned I had arthritis. I was really worried about my future ability to play tennis." The pain got worse. Concerns regarding his ability to walk replaced fears regarding his ability to play tennis.

Fortunately, he discovered a concerned, knowledgeable physician who placed him on anti-inflammatory therapy. Although delighted at his relatively prompt response to the medication, he was disappointed that only some of the pain and stiffness disappeared. His doctor's next suggestion — to play tennis — caught him by surprise. Wouldn't that make things worse? Much to Vic's delight, playing the sport he loved so much made his knees feel *better*. However, if he played more than four times a week, they felt worse, and, in fact, he would develop a noticeable limp. On the other hand, if he played less than two to three times a week the same thing would happen. He had discovered the exact amount of exercise necessary to control his arthritis. But remember — the amount of exercise best for this tennis legend may not be the best for you, so consult your doctor. (More on sports and arthritis in Chapter 14).

How successful has Vic's treatment been? He still plays in Grand Masters tournaments. In fact, at the age of 65 he reached the singles semifinals and won the doubles championship in his age group.

Now for a relatively easy way to take control of your arthritis.

When I'm tired it seems as if my joint pains are worse. Do you have any practical ways of dealing with this?

Fatigue is the curse of the arthritis sufferer, rest the blessing. In order to stress the importance of rest it is divided into different categories.

• *Joint rest* — This has been discussed in

Chapter 9 and entails everything from the principles of joint protection to using splints.

• *Emotional rest* — Stress may flare arthritis. This is further discussed below.

• *Physical rest* — This entails everything from taking a nap during the course of the day to relaxing in your favorite chair with your feet up. The balance between rest and activity will vary with the activity of your arthritis. Learn to pace yourself so you can complete your tasks without becoming fatigued. Do more when you're feeling well, less when you're not. Don't get overtired — it will only make your pain worse.

It seems that when I get a full night's sleep, my arthritis feels better. Is that my imagination?

No, it's not. The importance of sleep is becoming more and more appreciated. A good night's sleep used to be thought of as "useful." Now many physicians regard it as essential.

Many people with arthritis, or for that matter chronic pain of any type, develop poor sleep habits. A sound night's sleep appears to be associated with less joint discomfort and more energy. Conversely, lack of sleep often worsens the pain and increases fatigue. Thus a vicious cycle is created. The arthritis causes pain, which interferes with sleep, which makes the arthritis worse, which interferes with sleep even more, and so on, and so on . . .

Fibromyalgia is associated with sleep abnormalities. Recent research involving rheumatoid arthritis suggests that fatigue, which has classically been thought of as a manifestation of the disease process itself, may be due to sleep disruption as well.

If you are sleeping poorly, tell your doctor. It may be necessary to adjust your arthritis medicines. By reducing the arthritic pain, sleep is improved and the pain is further lessened. If you habitually awaken during the night, even if you think it is unrelated to arthritic pain, tell your doctor. Sometimes the sleep pattern is so severely disturbed that a more specific form of intervention, such as a sleeping pill or a sedative, is indicated. Don't self-medicate; don't buy something over the counter; don't take a relative's or friend's sleeping pills. Sleep is an extremely important factor, so tell your doctor what's going on and allow the doctor to help you.

The importance of the relationship between sleep and arthritic flare-ups is illustrated by a patient of mine who is a nurse. Despite having rheumatoid arthritis, Eleanor Conway functioned extremely well and rarely missed a day of work. Although her disease was under control most of the time, she'd occasionally suffer relatively severe flares, which were puzzling to both of us.

One day when she was in one of her flares I perused her record to determine when the last flare had taken place. Two months ago. The flare before — two months before that. The flares were all separated by a two-month period of time. Excitedly, I asked her what happened every two months. She changed shifts. We both sat silently for a few seconds, trying to understand the significance of our observations. Finally, it struck me.

"Do you have difficulty sleeping when your schedule changes?" I asked. She did. In fact, it often took her one to two weeks to adjust to the new schedule. Assuming this was the cause of her difficulty, I called the nursing supervisor and requested that my patient not have to change shifts. The request was granted.

That was five years ago. Since then Eleanor's sleep pattern has not been interrupted — and she hasn't had one flare of her arthritis!

Short of taking medication, do you have any hints for promoting good sleep? How much sleep do I need?

You need enough to make you feel well rested. There is nothing "magical" about eight hours of sleep a night. Some people require more, others less. Many people with rheumatoid arthritis require more than the average, so don't fight it, simply listen to your body. In fact, some patients with particularly active arthritis benefit from an afternoon nap.

A few hints to promote good sleep:

• Establish regular times to go to sleep and arise in the morning. Stick to the schedule — even on weekends. Many individuals who retire and awaken much later on weekends than during the week take two to three days to get back into a reasonable sleep rhythm.

• If you can't sleep, leave your bedroom, do something relaxing, and then return. Psychologically, the bed is a place for sleeping, not a place for tossing and turning while you worry that you can't sleep.

• Make the room as conducive to sleep as possible. If it's too light, get better drapes. If it's too warm, get a fan or air conditioner. If it's too noisy, play soothing music on the radio. If you have a favorite piece of peaceful music, play that regularly.

• If you're hungry before going to sleep, have a light snack. Don't go to bed hungry — or too full!

• Reduce or even eliminate caffeine, not just in the evening but all day if possible.

• Nicotine also serves as a stimulant — yet another reason to give up smoking!

• If you're not exercising, you will sleep better after you begin a program, another benefit of exercise.

• If everything fails, tell your doctor, who may want to put you on a longer acting anti-inflammatory drug with the hope it may get you through the night. What else can be done besides taking sleep medications? Deep breathing and relaxation exercises are often helpful. The sleep disturbance may be secondary to a depression — this is another avenue your physician may want to explore. Finally, antidepressants are often used in this situation, even if the patient is not depressed, as discussed in Chapter 8.

• Now some don'ts: don't use alcohol to help you sleep, and, as mentioned above, don't use an over-the-counter sleeping pill, and don't use someone else's sleeping pills. These can all lead to serious difficulties.

How about moving to a different climate as a way of getting better control of my arthritis?

Many people with arthritis feel better in a warm, dry climate, but if you don't live in such a place, the decision to move can be very difficult. You may feel more comfortable when you move, but it doesn't cure the arthritis. All aspects of such a move must be considered. Moves are stressful, and emotional, social, and financial factors must all be taken into consideration. The value of support from family and friends can't be overestimated.

If there are a number of reasons other than your arthritis to move, it is probably worthwhile. There is a good chance you will be disappointed if you move only because of your arthritis.

Discuss your move in detail with family members, friends, your physician, and any other health care professionals with whom you have been involved. Try to spend a month or two in the area you would like to relocate to before making a final decision.

We conclude this chapter with a few social

issues. The answers keep you — not family, friends, or business associates — in control of social situations.

How should I react when a family member or friend suggests a particular type of therapy?

Those around you are concerned with your well-being, but suggestions regarding your care can be annoying — especially if they are repetitious and without merit. Also, the suggestion may imply that you are not receiving the best possible care right now. This may make you defensive, especially if you have a good relationship with your doctor. On occasion, however, there may be some merit to the advice.

Don't be angry with the recommendations — remember, they're probably coming from a concerned individual. Thank the person for that concern and say you will discuss the situation with your doctor. If the suggestion sounds worthwhile, or if you want to satisfy your curiosity, do just that — ask your doctor about the suggestion. Sometimes it makes for an interesting conversation, and it may lead to something productive.

When my arthritis is active I find it difficult to shake hands. What do I do?

This simple ritual can be the cause of pain or embarrassment to the person with arthritis. One approach is simply to be honest and say you have arthritis. Another is to make good eye contact with the person you're meeting and nod your head. This shifts the focus away from the potential handshake. If the other person still offers a hand, either give a short, honest explanation or try one of the following.

If your right hand is bothering you but not your left, offer that hand in response — with or without an explanation, depending on the circumstances and how comfortable you feel. Or use both hands. With a little practice you will be able to do this comfortably, as the other person will usually lightly grip your hands. Finally, when appropriate, substitute a gentle hug or pat on the back. This will often extricate you from the situation.

When my rheumatoid arthritis is flaring I have to use a cane, sometimes even a walker. I'm just 40 years old and I get so embarrassed when people ask what's wrong I don't even want to go outside.

Remember that a lot of relatively young people have arthritis, and many of them have the same problem you do. Seek them out.

They can help you and you can help them. See how they handle similar situations.

Don't be a hostage to your arthritis. Let your doctor know when you're flaring and share your frustrations. This may lead to a change in your medication or physical therapy. Consider asking for a referral to an exercise class for patients with arthritis and perhaps a self-help group. The local chapter of the Arthritis Foundation may be helpful in this regard as well.

Don't be afraid to leave your home. That response is not healthy, from either a physical or an emotional perspective. Learn to deal with people who intrude on your privacy. Annie Potts sometimes uses a cane when her arthritis flares. She's a confident, self-possessed woman and she often finds that the people around her feel more uncomfortable about her using a cane than she does. When asked what's wrong with her, she simply says, "I'm fine, it's just arthritis." When someone asks you what's wrong, a straightforward answer like Annie Potts's is usually ideal. If someone goes on to express his sympathy, just thank him or say, "I'm doing fine." Pretty soon you will be, so get used to saying it.

11

Unconventional Therapy

Unconventional therapy is therapy that has not been scientifically shown to be effective. This does not always mean the treatment has not been tested, nor does it mean the results have not been positive. It simply means there haven't been enough tests to assure us the treatment is sound. For example, in this chapter the role of fish oil is discussed. Although a few studies have shown that this may be of value in the treatment of rheumatoid arthritis, a lot of work remains to be done before it can be classified as an accepted treatment option.

Of much more concern are treatments that have not been adequately studied and in essence are frauds. It has been estimated that between one and two billion dollars a year are spent on unproven remedies. There is more fraud involving arthritis than any other disease. Fraudulent remedies range from the harmless, such as wearing a copper bracelet, to the potentially dangerous. One hazardous gadget is the Detoxacolon, a pressurized enema that is said to rid the body of potentially noxious substances that supposedly cause arthritis. Not only do we lack scientific documentation of its efficacy, it may spread infection and even perforate the bowel wall, which could be fatal.

Why do some people persist in their belief that a certain form of therapy works, even if there is no scientific evidence to validate their perception? First, coincidences do happen, and since there are thirty-seven million arthritis sufferers in the United States there is a lot of opportunity for these to occur. Also, since arthritis is an extremely variable disease, it is easy to attach inappropriate significance to a new treatment. The arthritis may have been getting better anyway.

Second is the placebo response, which means you have a positive response to a treatment, such as the classical sugar pill, that should not work. This can be construed as an example of positive thinking — if you think something will work, it will. As many as one third of individuals exposed to a placebo will note improvement afterward.

The most common questions regarding unconventional therapy follow. Some answers may prove surprising — there may be something to these cures after all. But for the most part, if it is too good to be true, it probably isn't.

Is there anything I can add to my diet to improve my arthritis?

Patients have added a myriad of substances to their diets in the hope of controlling their arthritis. One of the most popular has been cod liver oil, the folk theory being that it helps lubricate joints. There is no evidence that this therapy is effective. But other types of fish oils are being studied, and preliminary findings indicate they may be of some benefit in the treatment of rheumatoid arthritis. Fish oils may also decrease the risk of heart disease. Eskimos have inspired research in this area, as they have a low incidence of both heart disease and arthritis and consume large amounts of fish. The answer is not that simple, however, as Eskimos generally lead healthy lives and get quite a bit of exercise.

Fish oil contains the polyunsaturated acids eicosapentaenoic acid (EPA) and docosahexaenoic acid (DHA), which are termed omega-3 fatty acids. It is these acids that may produce improvement in patients with rheumatoid arthritis. Although cod liver oil contains these acids, it is also rich in vitamins A and D (which can be dangerous if taken in large amounts) and cholesterol. Cod liver oil is therefore an inappropriate source of fish oil.

Although fish oil's effect on rheumatoid arthritis is seldom dramatic, it appears sufficiently safe to warrant being tried in addition to your regular treatment — not instead of it — if your physician so recommends. Common side effects include a gassy feeling in the stomach and a change in bowel habits, including the development of loose stools or constipation. Although there is some evidence that individuals consuming fish oils have a slightly impaired ability to clot blood, this is seldom if ever a practical consideration. Another potential drawback is the large number of pills, approximately fifteen to twenty, that must be taken daily, although the optimal dose is still unknown. In addition, the pills are quite expensive. Therefore, until further information is available, a reasonable approach is to increase consumption of fish rich in omega-3 fatty acids. These include oily, cold saltwater fish such as tuna, salmon, mackerel, and sardines. By taking this approach you can't lose. If further research fails to validate the somewhat beneficial effects noted thus far, you will have at least changed your diet for the better. If you insist on taking fish oil pills, double-check to be sure they contain low levels of saturated fats and no cholesterol.

Evening primrose oil has also been touted for its possible benefits to the arthritis sufferer.

The evening primrose is a yellow flower that opens at nightfall. It contains a polyunsaturated acid called gamma-linoleic acid, which is somewhat analogous to the fatty acids in fish oil. Dietary supplements of evening primrose oil have been given to research patients with rheumatoid arthritis, with results considerably less promising than those seen with fish oil supplementation.

Another suggested addition to the diet is calcium. The rationale is simple — bones are made of calcium, and when they are diseased it seems logical that they require more. Unfortunately, the addition of calcium to the diet does not affect the course of arthritis. On the other hand, some advocate the elimination of calcium from the diet since when tendons become inflamed they often become calcified; hence the conclusion that there is too much calcium in the diet. Again, this isn't true. The way inflamed tendons become calcified has nothing to do with the presence of extra calcium in the body.

Megadoses of vitamins have also been suggested as a cure for arthritis. There is no scientific validity for this stance, and this approach can in fact prove dangerous.

Other foods that have been extolled as treatments for arthritis include honey, vinegar, and various health foods, including alfalfa, yucca, and aloe vera. None has proven to be helpful.

When I explain to patients that the addition of various foodstuffs to their diets is unlikely to help their arthritis, most abandon the idea. A few, however, have persisted while still on conventional therapy, and a few insisted on treating themselves. With the possible exception of minor improvement after the addition of fish oil, I have never encountered a patient who responded to the addition of any food substance.

One particular patient comes to mind. He was sure the addition of cod liver oil to his diet would cure his osteoarthritic knee and insisted on pursuing this form of therapy before agreeing to be treated with anti-inflammatory drugs. His cure didn't work, and he was ultimately helped by a combination of medication and physical therapy. This man looked at least five years older than his actual age, was at least forty pounds overweight, reveled in steak, beer, and rich desserts, had a cholesterol level in the danger range, smoked two packs of cigarettes a day, and by his own admission was allergic to exercise. This is the man who wanted to treat his arthritis the natural way!

What about other kinds of doctors, such as chiropractors and osteopaths? Can they help?

In order to understand what chiropractors do, it is useful to understand their history. Chiropractic medicine was founded in 1895 by an Iowa grocer named D. D. Palmer. He believed that the nervous system controlled the body, and that all illnesses, including infections (he didn't believe in germs), could be cured by manipulating the nervous system.

After nerves exit the spinal cord they pass through an opening between two vertebral bodies. If the vertebral bodies aren't aligned properly, they can pinch the nerve. According to Palmer's theory, the nerve then misfires, and various diseases result as the body is deprived of a normal nerve supply. Palmer thought that by adjusting the spine, or manipulating it, he could take pressure off the involved areas and the patient would improve; all sorts of diseases — everything from diabetes to epilepsy — would get better. There is no evidence that Palmer's theory is true. Some chiropractors subscribe to Palmer's original theory. Many don't, restricting themselves to treating the conditions, such as joint problems, most likely to respond to their approach. Manipulation is all they have to offer, as they do not prescribe drugs or perform surgery.

What evidence is there that chiropractors help patients with musculoskeletal problems? Studies show that chiropractic adjustments provide quicker pain relief than a placebo — they are therefore better than nothing. After a few weeks, however, the benefits appear to cease. When manipulation is compared with massage techniques, it works more quickly. However, within six to seven weeks, the benefits appear equal.

Thus, if manipulation will help, it should be used early, and it makes little sense to use it for prolonged periods of time. Its effects may be transitory, and patients sometimes feel worse after a treatment session. There is no evidence it is useful in the treatment of chronic back pain.

Despite the perceived (and real) antagonism between physicians and chiropractors, many practitioners of the two disciplines recognize what the other has to offer and even refer patients to one another. It's important for all concerned to keep an open mind, especially when a patient's arthritis isn't improving.

My own experience with chiropractors indicates that they seem to be most worthwhile in dealing with acute cases. One particularly sobering experience I had with a chiropractor concerned a 23-year-old woman who had been experiencing severe knee pain for no apparent reason. She had originally been evaluated by an orthopedic surgeon, without a specific diagnosis being made. I saw her thereafter.

I was also unsure of the underlying problem but administered routine treatment because she was so uncomfortable. Nothing worked. The patient reached a point where she had a discernible limp. We were both growing desperate. I sent her to one of the finest orthopedic surgeons in Boston, a doctor who specialized in knee pain. He couldn't help. Finally, she asked me if she should see a chiropractor. I concurred, and suggested she come back thereafter. When she did, her pain was completely gone. It subsided after the first session with the chiropractor, disappeared after the fourth.

Elated (as well as surprised), I promptly called the chiropractor to find out what he thought the problem was and why his treatment worked. His simple answer amazed me. "I don't know," he said. "I don't know what her problem is, and I don't know why my treatment helped." At least he was honest — and he did help her.

Doctors of osteopathic medicine (osteopaths, or D.O.s) have training similar to traditional doctors — they prescribe medication and perform surgery — but they also believe in the importance of spinal manipulation and perform this procedure as well.

What about acupuncture?

Again we should be open-minded. Acupuncture occasionally appears capable of reducing the pain of arthritis but not the inflammation. Thus continued joint damage may ensue. There is no concrete evidence that it is an adequate treatment for arthritis, especially over the long run. Even in China other forms of therapy, including traditional Western approaches, are used to treat the arthritic patient.

In fact, there have been studies comparing sham acupuncture, in which needles are placed in the wrong place, with the real thing. Traditional acupuncture dictates that the needles be placed in very specific positions. There is often no difference in outcome between the two groups.

Despite this, acupuncture is sometimes helpful, and if you decide to try it, go to a bona fide acupuncturist, not a Western M.D. who isn't completely trained in the discipline.

Ironically, traditional Western medicine has incorporated techniques similar to those of chiropractic medicine and acupuncture. Physical therapists occasionally perform manipulation and also utilize acupressure and electrical stimulation, both of which are similar in theory to acupuncture (see Chapter 9). When physician audiences ask my opinion of acupuncture and chiropractors, I answer in the following way: When an acupuncturist treats a patient, many physicians call it quackery. When a physical therapist performs acupressure, it's advanced Western medicine. When a chiropractor performs manipulation, it's considered an invalid form of therapy. When a physical therapist does the same thing, it's good judgment.

In other words, as long as we are aware of the limitations of these unproven approaches, they may prove worthwhile in an occasional patient. But remember, they are not substitutes for a complete medical evaluation and should only be utilized with the advice and consent of your physician. I've seen too many patients who thought they had "routine" low back pain and went for acupuncture or spinal manipulation who were eventually discovered to have much more serious problems — including cancer.

Is there any benefit to yoga?

The word *yoga*, which literally means union, refers to a number of Hindu disciplines whose goal is to free the soul of earthly cares and merge it with God. This is accomplished in a number of ways, including meditation and the utilization of specific postures or exercises, which supposedly awaken various "energy centers" in the body. Some of these exercises are similar to range-of-motion exercises taught by physical therapists. Yoga exercises are performed slowly while practicing deep breathing techniques. Force and stress are not involved, and there are no bouncing, jerky motions. In a sense they are the opposite of high-impact aerobic exercises, which are good for keeping in shape but do not offer any benefit to your joints. Although yoga appears to be rather safe on the whole, some of the advanced positions can put extra stress on the joints and should be avoided.

Patients with arthritis often find the exercises beneficial and claim that yoga also provides a means of relaxing and reducing stress. Juliet Prowse is a major proponent of yoga. She finds it helpful for her joints as well as a wonderful stress reducer. When not on the road she attends classes two to three times a week. Donna McKechnie is also a major advocate of yoga and thinks it is one of the factors that improved her rheumatoid arthritis. Although not yet scrutinized by Western statistical analysis, yoga appears sufficiently safe and potentially helpful to warrant giving it a try if you are so inclined. It is not a substitute for a traditional medical and physical therapy approach but can be used to supplement them. Indeed, some patients carry over the principles of yoga to their physical therapy programs and claim to be much the better for the combination.

I heard that DMSO is a good treatment for arthritis. What is it, and is this true?

DMSO, or dimethyl sulfoxide, is a drug widely used in veterinary medicine. There is no evidence that it is anything but a mild pain reliever. It is usually available in a veterinary strength not intended for human use. Skin rashes, headache, nausea, and diarrhea can result from its use. It also produces a garliclike taste in the mouth. It is applied topically and given intravenously. Clinics have sprung up that administer this drug. Patients are encouraged to return frequently, as often as three or four times a week, and often at great expense. There is nothing to suggest this approach is helpful; in fact, it is potentially harmful because side effects may result and more reliable treatments may be ignored.

Is there anything I can rub on my joints to make them feel better?

As discussed in Chapter 9, the application of heat and cold is routine in the treatment of arthritis, both in the physical therapist's office and as part of a home treatment program. Both modalities make joints feel better. Heat also relaxes muscles, and cold may reduce inflammation.

On the other hand, rub-on balms and creams are rarely if ever prescribed, as there is little scientific evidence to support their use. This represents the traditional view taken by most rheumatologists. However, these preparations have not been extensively evaluated and many patients find them helpful. The first rub-on preparation was invented in the late 1800s by a French pharmacist named Bengue. It was introduced in the United States in 1898 and is still available, although the name has been anglicized to Ben-Gay®. Many similar preparations have been introduced over the years. They probably work by irritating the skin, thus generating some heat. The skin discomfort may take your mind off your joint pain, and the small amount of heat generated may have a positive effect as well. As with any form of therapy, there may be a placebo effect. In fact, one study compared the active ingredient of a number of these preparations with a placebo in the treatment of osteoarthritis of the knee and found no difference between them.

Some of these products contain salicylates, which are contained in aspirin products, and it is implied that the salicylate is absorbed into the joint where it exerts a local anti-inflammatory effect. This does not appear to be the case. If you are allergic to aspirin or other salicylates, you may be allergic to some of these preparations as well. Therefore, don't use them without checking with your doctor.

These products are probably harmless, so if you think they make you feel better there's no harm in continuing. The major exception is if you rely on them to the extent that you don't seek appropriate medical care.

If you do use these preparations, don't use heating pads. Heat enhances the absorption of menthol, the active ingredient in many of these preparations, and this can lead to tissue damage. Also, some of these compounds give off a strong odor, which many find unpleasant. If you use these products frequently, especially during the day, you may ultimately fail to recognize their smell. Unfortunately, the same can't always be said for the people around you!

Radiation is used to treat other serious diseases. Can it be used to treat arthritis?

X-ray therapy directed to the spine was once used to treat ankylosing spondylitis but was abandoned, in part because of the subsequent development of malignancies.

More recently, radiation directed to the lymph nodes has been used to treat rheumatoid arthritis. The rationale behind this is that rheumatoid arthritis is an autoimmune disease. Since lymph nodes represent an essential part of the immune system, rheumatoid arthritis may improve by temporarily "poisoning" the immune system.

Results of studies thus far have been promising, as many subjects have noted long-term improvement of their arthritis following treatment. On occasion this has lasted more than one year. On the other hand, the side effects of radiation therapy are often unpleasant, including, among others, nausea, vomiting, decreased appetite, and hair loss. These problems disappear after cessation of therapy. A more serious problem is the development of infections, as the positive effects of the immune system are diminished along with the negative. Lymph node radiation remains an experimental form of therapy for only the most severe cases of rheumatoid arthritis.

My neighbor went to Mexico to have his arthritis treated. He felt better for a while, but then the medicine wore off. Is it worth the trip?

A number of arthritis clinics have sprouted

along the Texas border. They utilize drugs such as cortisone and phenylbutazone, both of which have extremely strong anti-inflammatory effects but are potentially dangerous and require meticulous follow-up, as well as drugs that have been inadequately tested. A number of people have become seriously ill as a result of this unsupervised therapy; others have died.

A word to the wise . . .

What about copper bracelets?

This question can be answered succinctly. They are of no value whatsoever. Blood levels of copper in patients with rheumatoid arthritis are higher than normal, so even on purely theoretical grounds the bracelet is worthless.

Those of you who still think you can successfully treat arthritis by dietary manipulation will point to the above observation and suggest eliminating copper from the diet. However, the increased copper level is a result of the inflammatory reaction, not of nutritional aberrations, and cannot be corrected by dietary control.

Every year I go to a spa and my arthritis improves. Is it my imagination? Should I keep going?

This question usually comes from my European patients, who are used to this type of approach. In fact, many of them insist on returning to a spa yearly. They usually come back improved, and the improvement often lasts for a number of months.

Upon close analysis it becomes apparent that health spas do more than expose their proponents to mineral springs. For example, they advocate and provide a healthy, well-balanced diet. Exercise classes are available and often mandatory. Various types of physical therapy are provided. By definition, the patient is removed from home and family pressures.

So it's not surprising that most people return from spas feeling refreshed. But I doubt it's the mineral water that's doing it.

I read that bee stings can make arthritis better. Is it worth it?

No, it's not worth it. Rarely, patients with arthritis who have been stung by bees report a temporary improvement, no doubt as a result of the production of various hormones that have an anti-inflammatory effect. Enterprising individuals have capitalized on this and in essence sold bee stings for a profit. Some who tout this form of therapy claim it takes hundreds, even thousands of stings to really make a difference. This therapy is potentially dangerous and has no proven scientific merit. Also, you may be allergic to bee venom and not know it; an allergic reaction could have dire consequences.

Speaking of hormones, the final question in this section involves one of the most popular unproven remedies . . .

Someone told me sex can help arthritis. Is this true?

Believe it or not, it can — but only temporarily. Sex stimulates the production of various hormones such as cortisone and adrenaline. Some of these substances have a natural anti-inflammatory effect and can reduce pain for a little while.

I first became aware of this after one of my patients returned from a Florida vacation feeling much better than before she left. When I asked her to explain her improvement, she said, "The warm weather, not having to think about my job, and sex." Regular sexual relations with a newfound lover resulted in a clearcut improvement in her joint inflammation, which lasted for hours to days at a time.

You can draw your own conclusions — but remember, it's not a substitute for conventional therapy.

★ ★ ★

From a practical perspective, how can unproven remedies be recognized? If a treatment is said to be successful for all forms of arthritis, it should be viewed skeptically. Remember, there are over one hundred kinds of arthritis, and it is unlikely that one remedy is good for all of them. Be especially skeptical about claims of a cure. Be skeptical when a treatment has a limited number of advocates, especially when a lot of publicity is attached to that therapy. Be even more cautious if the proponents of a new treatment find it necessary to lambast conventional medicine. Question the evidence that the treatment works — especially if it consists of individual case histories or testimonials or a single study. A number of large studies are required to prove that a treatment outcome is not due to chance or a placebo effect.

Remember — as previously stated — if a treatment sounds too good to be true, it probably isn't.

12

Taking Charge of
Your Attitude

Faith and knowledge lean largely upon
each other in the practice of medicine.
— PETER MERE LATHAM

How important is your attitude when you
have arthritis? Some researchers believe it
may be more important than the illness itself.
For example, assume there are two patients
with the same disease, similar in severity,
receiving the same treatment. One does well,
the other poorly. Why is this? Investigators
have attempted to answer this question by
examining groups of patients with arthritis.
After determining the extent of the illness
in each of the study participants, they have
assessed a number of psychological factors,
including depression, anxiety, and feelings of
helplessness. They have concluded that the
amount of pain and disability experienced by
individual patients is not explained by joint
damage alone and is significantly influenced
by their attitudes and emotional state.

It may surprise you to learn that there is nothing new about this idea. In fact Hippocrates, the father of medicine, recognized the importance of emotions and their relationship to disease almost 2500 years ago. Classical psychology teaches us that there are a number of normal emotional reactions to the development of arthritis. Initially there may be denial that the illness is present. This can turn into anger, anxiety, and depression before the person comes to terms with the problem. This represents a "textbook" sequence of events, which may or may not take place in an individual patient. However, you should be aware of these reactions so you can recognize them. In many instances only depression or anger will be obvious.

Denial is a psychological defense mechanism designed to protect the individual from threatening information. People often utter the words "I can't believe it" when hearing a piece of bad news. When this truly occurs — that is, when they don't allow themselves to fully comprehend what is happening to them — denial is taking place. Denial usually occurs early in the illness, especially when symptoms first appear and the person shies away from going to the doctor. However, it can occur at any time, often when the arthritis flares.

It is a normal reaction and is seldom harmful unless it leads patients to overexert themselves or not take their medication. Patients with diabetes often exhibit denial when they refuse to watch their diets. The same is true for people with heart disease who refuse to recognize their limitations.

There are many reasons for depression. These include pain, fatigue, stress, and fear of loss — loss of a loved one, lifestyle, or body image. Inability to express anger may also lead to depression. Although depression and anger are considered normal responses to the development of arthritis, that doesn't make them any easier to tolerate. In fact, they can heighten your response to pain.

Stress can also worsen your perception of pain. Just as the previously discussed reactions are normal, so are the reactions to stress. But if your joints hurt more, that's no consolation. When the brain perceives stress it sends out a number of messages to the rest of your body. The result is increased levels of various hormones, an increased heart and breathing rate, increased blood pressure, a marked increase in blood flow to the arms and legs, and increased muscle tension. The stress reaction was initially intended to protect our bodies from physical harm. In modern days, however, most stress results from emotional or mental challenges. A proper dose of stress can improve performance, as during an athletic event or when taking an examination. If the stress is dealt with in a positive fashion, the body restores itself. Should this not be the case, or if the stress is more constant, stress-related tension builds up and a number of changes may take place.

The symptoms of stress are numerous and include fatigue, anxiety, an exaggerated sense of worry, nervousness, increased muscle tension, appetite changes, indigestion and stomach aches, difficulty sleeping, and decreased libido. A number of immunological changes occur as well.

We have already established that arthritis is not *caused* by stress (see Chapter 4), but stress can certainly aggravate the situation. The increased muscle tension associated with stress can increase joint pain. Arthritis can also flare because of the immunological changes that accompany stress. Increased pain can lead to depression, which leads to more stress, more pain — and a very unhealthy cycle is created.

Why do we tolerate stress so poorly? An interesting postulate has been voiced by Dr. Robert Eliot, a cardiologist, who is director of the Institute of Stress Medicine in Denver, Colorado, and the author of *Is It Worth Dying*

For? Dr. Eliot points out that the physiological changes that occur as a result of stress have not significantly evolved over the years, so the changes that occurred in a caveman when he fought a saber-toothed tiger are virtually identical to those that occur today in a businessman struggling to meet a deadline, a student preparing for an examination, or a parent trying to take care of more than one screaming child at the same time. But whereas a caveman might only have to fight a saber-toothed tiger a few times in his lifetime, Eliot's studies show that as many as seventeen percent of us "are fighting tigers 40 or 50 times a day." Although Eliot's research specifically addressed the issue of blood pressure elevation and its relationship to stress, a number of immunological studies show that fighting those tigers is detrimental to arthritis as well.

What can be done to improve the emotional state and attitudes of patients with arthritis and to keep stress at a minimum? These issues are discussed in response to the following questions.

Doctors have a responsibility to educate their patients. Some patients like to know as much as possible about their illness. Others appear totally uninterested. One of the latter expressed her feelings about her illness and then asked the following question.

I'm only 28 years old and I already have arthritis. I'm so disgusted I don't even want to talk about it. It's bad enough I have it — why should I have to know anything more about it?

There are a number of reasons why patients should be educated regarding their disease. Those who understand the rationale behind their treatment are more likely to follow their physicians' and therapists' suggestions. For example, once they understand that their usual daily activities do not move their joints through a normal range of motion, they are more likely to do their range-of-motion exercises. Once they understand why it is necessary to take anti-inflammatory medication on a regular basis, they will be more likely to do so.

As discussed in Chapter 4, people do better when they think they can do something to influence their disease. The more helpless they feel, the worse they usually do. Knowledge brings about a feeling of control, a feeling that you have the power to influence your illness.

A very practical way of being educated is to attend an arthritis self-help course. Ask your physician about them or call the local chapter of the Arthritis Foundation. These courses are usually quite comprehensive, covering both theoretical and practical aspects of arthritis. Patients who complete these courses usually feel more in control and, as a result, exercise more often and report less pain. In fact, gaining a sense of control may be of even greater benefit than the actual information learned in the course.

If you still "just don't want to know" about your arthritis, you may be experiencing denial or anger, the psychological reactions discussed above. It is important that you recognize this so you don't do something to hurt yourself, such as over-exercising or missing doses of medication. Otherwise there's not much to be done for denial. In fact, most psychologists believe there should not be any attempts to confront denial unless absolutely necessary. In time, denial usually dissipates, and people ultimately acquire additional information at their own pace.

Anger, on the other hand, can build up and lead to depression. The best way of dealing with anger is to express your emotions. Talk to your doctor, a family member, or a friend — anyone with whom you feel comfortable. If the feeling persists, ask your physician about referral to a psychologist or social worker. You can also try talking into a tape recorder or keeping a diary. Anything you do to provide an outlet for your emotions will serve you well. That way you control your emotions, not vice versa.

After I feel particularly stressed, my arthritis flares. Is there anything I can do to prevent that from happening?

There are a number of ways to reduce stress. Start by identifying the causes of stress in your life, as illustrated by the following two stories.

Maureen Kent, a 28-year-old woman with rheumatoid arthritis, rarely complained about her joints. Her arthritis was well controlled by an anti-inflammatory medication and a vigorous exercise program to which she religiously adhered. So when her arthritis flared I was more than a bit puzzled. Reluctantly, I increased her medication, the flare subsided, and the dose was then decreased. This continued to occur at regular intervals — approximately every eight to ten weeks.

As soon as I realized there was a pattern I asked her what occurred at that time interval. At first she said nothing did. Then she thought for a few moments and realized the time frame coincided with deadlines at work. Although she admitted the deadlines were stressful, she made no connection between the flares of her arthritis and her work stress — yet when we examined the dates of the flares, they coincided perfectly with the deadlines!

Although Maureen still wasn't convinced, we decided on a little experiment. The main reason for the stress, she concluded, was that she waited until the last minute before preparing her work. She reluctantly agreed to make a schedule for herself so she would finish her work at least two to three days before it was due. The result — no more flares of her arthritis.

The second example is that of Alice Titus, a young woman with rheumatoid arthritis who was going through a particularly stressful stage in her marriage. Almost every time she had an argument with her husband, her arthritis would flare — usually within thirty-six hours. They recognized their problem and went into counseling. Within a relatively brief period of time, their arguments decreased in number and intensity, and so did the flares.

Neither of these patients was cured by reducing her stress. Both continued to require routine therapy. But both were clearly improved by virtue of the changes in their lives.

Your arthritis may also be worsened by periodic stressful events, so you might want to apply this tactic to your own life. Identify the factors that increase your stress — even if you don't recognize an association with your arthritis — and do something about it!

Here are a few practical suggestions for reducing stress and anxiety.

• Modify your activities. Make a concerted effort to identify stress. Keep a log, and then look back to determine the main sources of difficulty.

• Exercise. When your work day is done (whether that is in or outside the home), do something physical. By engaging in physical activity later in the day, you defuse the tensions you've accumulated and thus may get more benefit from an exercise program in the afternoon or evening than in the morning. Once you get in good condition, however, the benefits of exercise will have long-range effects, and the time of day you exercise will become less important.

• Take advantage of nature. Go to a park on a warm day, walk on the beach or in the grass. In the wintertime, relax in front of a fireplace.

• Find a hobby. Hobbies provide opportunities to lose yourself and can be incredibly relaxing.

• Pets, especially dogs, have been shown by many studies to reduce stress. Juliet Prowse is one of Hollywood's biggest animal lovers. She presently has four dogs, and walks them at least twice a day. They have been trained to walk by her side, without a leash. Ironically, one of them, a golden retriever, just had hip surgery for arthritis. By the way, the walks are not a token trip up the street and back. They average approximately two miles, providing Juliet with exercise as well as time to be with her pets.

Raising tropical fish can also be a soothing hobby. In fact, studies have shown that viewing tropical fish can be associated with a decrease in blood pressure, which is associated with decreased stress. Photographer Alfred Eisenstaedt raised tropical fish throughout much of his life and has found them a great source of relaxation. In his 90s, he found their care a bit burdensome and substituted a terrarium, which he finds equally comforting.

The value of pets and plants is accentuated if you have at least part of the responsibility for their care.

• Listen to music. Lie down in a darkened room and listen to soothing music. This has always been a favorite of Alfred Eisenstaedt.

• Allocate a period of time for yourself to do what you want. If you are extremely busy, schedule the time, much as you would an appointment.

• Work on being as honest with yourself and others as possible. If you need help with something, admit it and ask for it. If you're having trouble with school or job, make the necessary modifications.

This approach made an enormous difference to one of my patients with rheumatoid arthritis. Patricia Tresh had always been an independent person, and when she developed arthritis at the age of 35 it had a devastating effect. She simply could not ask others for help. Activities she should have avoided resulted in increased pain, and as her pain increased she became more and more depressed. She finally agreed to go to an arthritis support group, where she learned how to ask for assistance without embarrassment. Simple things, like asking the waiter delivering her room service breakfast to open the jar of jelly, made a big difference. A lesson she learned, and in fact asked me to put in this book, is that it is more damaging to keep trying something and failing than to ask for help.

• If you feel depressed, realize that you are

responsible for how you feel. This should enable you to play a more active role in improving your emotional state. Try to force yourself to do the things you normally enjoy. Usually you'll feel better afterward.

• Call a friend or a relative. Express your feelings, and don't be afraid to cry. Consider asking for professional help. Tell your physician if you are not doing well emotionally — an extra appointment to talk about emotional issues may prove beneficial. Your doctor may suggest counseling or perhaps a medication to reduce stress or depression. Your medication may even be playing a role, and your physician may suggest changing it.

• When people are stressed, they may resort to what they regard as short-term solutions, such as drugs and alcohol. These are long-term problems, not short-term solutions. In the long run they increase your stress and depression.

What can you do if these relatively simple suggestions are ineffective? I spoke with Dr. Joan Borysenko, who began her career as a cell biologist, became a clinical psychologist, and emerged as an expert on stress and a bestselling author. Her book *Minding the Body, Mending the Mind* has proven helpful to thousands of readers.

Dr. Borysenko emphasizes the importance of social support, especially from family and friends, as a stress reducer. "The first buffer against stress is the number of people you can depend on," she says. She is quick to point out, however, that even if you are fortunate enough to have a loving family, you will probably still benefit from a support group. Some families, no matter how well intentioned, have a smothering effect on the person with arthritis. The support group supplements the family and meets additional emotional needs. Support groups teach people to be more resourceful, which correlates with an increased ability to deal with problems such as arthritis. They put their members back in control.

Dr. Borysenko also thinks most people can benefit from relaxation techniques designed to reduce stress. These methods give people a sense of control and hope and involve a concept that is new to most people. Dr. Borysenko says, "People can learn to take responsibility for the consequences of their emotions. They can learn that they have a choice."

Dr. Herbert Benson of Harvard Medical School has done much of the pioneering work in the field of stress reduction. He is the author of a number of books on the subject, and his first book title, *The Relaxation Response,* has become a widely used term to describe the physiological consequences of stress reduction.

According to Dr. Benson, stress reduction is a valuable way to reduce the perception of pain. He views pain as a vicious cycle. Pain leads to anxiety and stress, which leads to more pain, which leads to more anxiety and stress, and so on. These reactions are associated with increased blood pressure, heart rate, rate of breathing, and muscle tension — in other words, all the elements of a stress response.

Dr. Benson suggests a specific technique to reduce stress, namely the repetition of a word, sound, or phrase in time with your breathing, as you exhale. He suggests words and phrases such as *peace, love, the Lord is my shepherd,* and *shalom.* This should be done in a quiet area for ten to twenty minutes twice a day.

This leads to what is now termed the relaxation response. The person becomes calm, less anxious, less depressed, and less hostile. Blood pressure, heart rate, and breathing rate all go down. Muscle tension is reduced, and pain often subsides. Although the exercise is done only twice daily, many people feel these effects throughout the day.

This sounds good, and it often is. But will it always reduce arthritic pain? Unfortunately the answer is no, but even if it doesn't reduce your discomfort, there is a good chance you will experience less anxiety and depression.

The repetition of a word in time with your breathing is only one relaxation technique. Others include simple deep breathing exercises, self-hypnosis, biofeedback, and imagery or visualization. Prayer can reduce stress. Some people visualize calm scenes, such as oceans or mountains. Actress Jane Withers visualized herself singing and dancing and found this to be a very valuable tool.

Finally, remember that *your emotions did not create your arthritis, and it isn't your fault if you don't get better.* Even though the methods described above may work for some people, they don't for others. If they don't work for you, it's not because you have a bad attitude. Solutions to complex problems involving the mind and body are very personal. Your solution may not be obvious, but with perseverance, hope, and a lot of hard work, it will come in time.

Exercise is a popular and effective way of reducing stress and making you feel better about yourself. But what happens if it doesn't work?

I decided to exercise to help my arthritis and reduce my stress, but it hasn't helped. Why is that?

Just as performing relaxation techniques twice a day can be helpful throughout the entire day, exercise can have a far-reaching effect as well. In fact, it is beginning to appear that exercise and relaxation techniques may have similar effects on stress levels. Even more benefit occurs when you combine the two. When people meditate or use an appropriate relaxation technique while exercising, the exercise becomes more efficient and less tiring. The best way to work out your body is to relax your mind at the same time.

The individual who asked the above question chose swimming as her form of exercise because she reasoned it was best for her arthritis. Swimming is indeed an excellent form of exercise, but this woman did not enjoy it and as a result it actually increased her anxiety level because she never felt truly comfortable in the water. Before she developed arthritis she loved to do low-impact aerobics, and I suggested she go back to it. She's now learned to relax while exercising and has reaped enormous benefit from her new exercise program.

Norman Cousins cured his arthritis by utilizing the powers of his mind. How did he do it?

Norman Cousins's contributions to the field

of stress research are unique. The victim of an acute arthritic disease in 1964, he utilized what he thought were the powers of the mind to help overcome his illness. His first-person account in *Anatomy of an Illness* had an enormous impact on both the lay and medical communities. Fascinated by the relationship between the mind and body, Cousins left his long-standing editorship of the *Saturday Review* to join the faculty of the School of Medicine at the University of California at Los Angeles. His book *Head First, the Biology of Hope* is the culmination of ten years of research into this engrossing but elusive area.

The following is a brief description of Dr. Cousins's experiences. When conventional approaches failed to control his arthritis he turned to alternate treatments. Convinced that "negative emotions" were harmful, Cousins speculated that "positive emotions" would prove beneficial. Accordingly, he viewed humorous television shows such as "Candid Camera" and Marx Brothers movies. He soon discovered that ten minutes of laughter allowed him up to two hours of pain-free sleep. Slowly and steadily, over a number of years, he got better. He attributed his improvement to a cleansing of his mind, which subsequently allowed his body to heal.

Did Cousins really cure his illness, or was

it a coincidence that he went into remission? Certainly patients with similar diseases go into spontaneous remissions. Did he help that process along? Would it have happened anyway?

As of now we cannot answer these questions with certainty, but we have learned that positive attitudes can effect various biochemical changes within the body and that negative attitudes can adversely affect our health.

I spoke with Cousins and asked him to put his personal experiences and research into perspective. He felt badly that some people had misinterpreted the intent of *Anatomy of an Illness*. "If I had to do the whole thing over again, I'd be sure people didn't come away with the impression I was trying to advocate a specific type of therapy to the exclusion of others. People can't simply 'ha ha' their way out of a bad thing. My approach is integral to, not a substitute for, other care."

In other words, he wasn't advocating the refusal of conventional therapy. What he was advocating is an acknowledgment that we can help the body by helping the mind. "Any serious disease has a tendency to produce depression. The depression can then exacerbate the disease. The wise physician realizes he treats only half the patient if he treats the body, only half if he treats the mind."

We've come a long way in our understanding of the mind and its relationship to disease, but we have an even longer way to go. There are few who would say that stress causes arthritis, but it almost certainly worsens it. As a corollary, the reduction of stress will probably be beneficial. There are many ways to reduce stress. One is by laughter.

This is not a new concept. In 1737 Matthew Green wrote, "Laugh and be well." It took over 250 years to prove he was right.

13

Sexuality and Arthritis

Arthritis is a pervasive disease, affecting not just the specific joints involved, but numerous other physical and emotional aspects of your life and the lives of those around you. One of the most sensitive of these aspects is sexuality, still an embarrassing topic throughout much of our society. Ideally, you should be able to discuss this subject comfortably with your doctor, but this is not always the case. Physicians are often guilty of not bringing it up, even more guilty for not picking up on their patients' cues. If the doctor feels comfortable talking about sexuality, the patient may not. Add it all up and you get a lot of poor communication.

This chapter is meant to serve as a catalyst, a stimulus to discuss your own concerns with your spouse or lover and an interested professional if necessary. If your doctor is uncomfortable discussing these issues, ask to be referred to someone who is not. Nurses, social workers, psychologists, and psychiatrists are all usually helpful in this regard.

Ever since I developed arthritis I've lost interest in sex. My marriage is deteriorating. Is there anything I can do?

According to noted psychologist and syndicated columnist Dr. Joyce Brothers, there are specific reasons for a decline in sexual interest in people with arthritis. The first is physical pain, which is discussed below. Second, patients with arthritis may be depressed. This decreases *libido*, or sexual desire. Chronic illnesses such as rheumatoid arthritis may also decrease sexual drive, especially when the disease is quite active. Finally, changes in physical appearance may make you feel less desirable, which also decreases libido. The good news is that arthritis per se seldom has an effect on the sexual organs.

These problems can all be dealt with, but it's difficult to do it on your own. That's why Dr. Brothers recommends that the patient and spouse discuss them with a physician or other appropriate health care professional.

Let's talk about these issues in more depth.

Depression is a normal reaction to the development of arthritis, but it doesn't last forever. It often occurs early in the disease and returns when the disease flares. Once the condition is accepted, emotional and physical energy can be rechanneled in a more positive fashion.

In addition, as the arthritis is treated and improves, depression often diminishes. Sexual interest usually then increases. Dr. Brothers emphasizes that when people with arthritis are going through particularly bad times, it is important that they understand their sex lives are not over but simply on hold. This simple realization is often quite encouraging to both partners.

If you are concerned about your body image, don't suffer in silence. Discuss it with your partner. It's often not the issue you've made it in your own mind, but the only way you are going to know this is by discussing it. In my practice I frequently encounter patients who are extremely upset by changes in their physical appearance, mostly in their hands. The majority of these individuals are women. It is often striking how minor these changes really are, and patients brighten when this is pointed out to them. They initially think I'm simply trying to make them feel better, but I explain that they are more sensitive to changes in their body than anyone else.

Part of your depression and decreased libido may be in response to what you perceive as your partner's decreased interest in lovemaking. That in turn may be caused by a fear of hurting you, which is seldom realistic. This problem can usually be worked out as discussed in the question below and is a perfect example of how open and honest communication can improve one's love life.

If you do have disabilities, others often automatically assume you have no interest in sexual relations. This is pure and simple prejudice and is groundless. In fact, love-making is important under these circumstances as it increases intimacy and enhances one's confidence. But no one will know how you feel unless you talk about it.

As noted in Chapter 11, love-making may make your arthritis feel better because of hormonal changes or the production of endorphins, which are substances our bodies manufacture to decrease pain. This is certainly an irony — most people are concerned that sexual intimacy makes arthritis worse, yet the opposite is probably true!

During times when you are not interested in love-making, it is important to discuss this. Don't just turn away, which may compound any emotional problems that may be developing with your lover. Find other ways to show your love and affection. A simple act such as holding hands can result in enormous intimacy under the right circumstances.

Finally, always consider the possibility that decreased sexual desires may have other causes. For example, postpartum depression may be decreasing your libido. Breast-feeding may alter sexual desire, either decreasing or increasing it. The same can be said for birth control pills.

Ever since I found out I have arthritis I'm afraid to make love, and my husband thinks he'll hurt me. Is that true? Is there anything to be concerned about?

There are no specific reasons to avoid love-making, but there are some caveats. The main deterrent to love-making is pain. This makes sense when one considers that areas frequently attacked by arthritis, such as the knee, hip, and low back, are stressed during the act of intercourse. It is therefore easy to understand why the traditional missionary position for making love can be very uncomfortable if the woman has arthritis in her hips or the man in his arms or knees. Experiment with different positions. Consider your most comfortable postures while lying down and try to adapt your love-making positions to them. Many women with arthritis find it most comfortable to be on top during intercourse, but that doesn't mean it's best for you.

As discussed above, communication is the key. Just as patients often feel uncomfortable discussing issues of sexuality with their physicians and vice versa, lovers often avoid discussing the topic with one another. Talk to your partner. If a position is uncomfortable, don't put up with the pain. Experiment, and don't give up.

I still enjoy love-making, but I get frustrated when I'm tired or my joints ache. Do you have any practical suggestions?

Indeed, there are practical ways of dealing with this situation, the most important of which is to plan your sexual activity. Although this may be alien to your way of thinking, try to be open-minded.

How do you do this?

• Pick a time during the course of the day when you usually feel better. For example, patients with rheumatoid arthritis are usually stiff in the morning, and stiffness may return later in the day. Therefore make love between those two times.

• Schedule your love-making to coincide with the peak activity of your medication.

• Treat your love-making as a form of exercise, which it really is. Take a warm bath beforehand to relax you and your muscles. Do range-of-motion exercises as well.

• Schedule love-making for days that are not otherwise laden with strenuous activities. For example, if you schedule it for a particular afternoon, don't vacuum the house that morning.

Although it was previously stated that arthritis does not interfere with sexuality per se, there may be an exception in some individuals.

Since I developed arthritis I've noticed a problem with vaginal dryness. Could there be a relationship?

Decreased vaginal lubrication can result from a number of factors, including the normal changes that accompany aging and the use of various medications. The latter includes some of the drugs used to treat infertility and endometriosis. Various types of arthritis may be associated with vaginal dryness, especially if Sjogren's syndrome (see Chapter 5) is present. Just as Sjogren's syndrome results in dryness in the mouth and eyes, it can result in vaginal dryness as well.

Discuss the problem with your doctor. One solution may be to use a lubricant such as K-Y jelly. Avoid petroleum-based products, which are not water-soluble. They may block pores and possibly lead to infections. Various types of hormone creams may be suggested as well.

I want to have a child. Does that mean I have to stop my medication?

You must discuss this issue with your doctor and spouse. If you decide to get pregnant, your doctor will discontinue as many medications as possible. All remission-inducing agents should be stopped and pregnancy avoided for at least one menstrual cycle, perhaps more, as your physician advises. This is important for all remission-inducing agents, but especially for methotrexate, which may cause fetal abnormalities or death. If an unanticipated pregnancy occurs while on a remission-inducing agent, call your doctor immediately.

Usually you can continue taking anti-inflammatory medications while you're trying to become pregnant, although some physicians prefer switching to acetaminophen.

Once conception occurs, your physician will prefer that you take as little medication as possible. On the other hand, you have to be able to continue to function, and this may require an anti-inflammatory drug or acetaminophen, again at the discretion of your doctor.

Fortunately, pregnancy brings on hormonal changes that usually result in adequate control of arthritis, so many women do not have to take medications during their pregnancy. The arthritis often returns after the baby is born. At that time the appropriate medications can be resumed.

If you remain on anti-inflammatory drugs and have been unable to conceive, discuss the possibility of stopping them with your doctor. It is theoretically possible that these medications may be interfering with your ability to become pregnant. Although it is unlikely, it may be worth a try. Acetaminophen can be substituted for pain control.

Do men have to stop taking medication when the decision is made to have a baby?

For the most part medications the male partner is taking do not appear to decrease chances of conception or create problems in the child. An exception is methotrexate, and you should stop taking this drug at least three months prior to attempting conception.

Men should also discuss these issues with their physician as there may be additional exceptions.

The next questions discuss various aspects

of pregnancy as it relates to arthritis.

Can I exercise while I'm pregnant?

The answer to this question is a qualified yes. The time to get serious about your exercise program is before you get pregnant, not after. If you have not been exercising, pregnancy is the wrong time to start.

Use your planned pregnancy as a stimulus to exercise. Learn range-of-motion exercises and begin a conditioning program, as advised by your physician and physical therapist. Continue the exercises during the pregnancy. Do what you're used to doing. Do not increase the difficulty of your program. Take particular pains to avoid sustained aerobic exercises unless they've been part of your prior program. These exercises shunt extra blood to the muscles at the expense of other areas of your body, including the uterus. Serious problems with the pregnancy could ensue. Swimming is an excellent exercise to continue throughout much of your pregnancy. The buoyancy of the water reduces the stress on your joints. It also provides an excellent aerobic workout. Finally, try not to gain too much extra weight. It puts additional stress on your joints both during and after the pregnancy. Your obstetrician can help guide you in this area.

I want to breast-feed my baby. Can I still take medication?

Most medications used to treat arthritis are passed by the mother's milk to the baby and should not be taken during breast-feeding. An exception to this appears to be ibuprofen, which is undetectable in breast milk at daily doses of 2400 mg or less. However, don't take this or any other drug while breast-feeding without discussing it with your physician.

During my pregnancy my hands started to get numb. Even though I have arthritis in my hands, I never had that symptom before. What is causing the numbness?

This is a common complaint among pregnant women and is usually caused by carpal tunnel syndrome, which is discussed in Chapter 5. Carpal tunnel syndrome is associated with a number of arthritic conditions, including rheumatoid arthritis. It may occur in pregnancy in the absence of arthritis because of weight gain.

The syndrome also may occur in the postpartum period, when excessive use of the hands associated with carrying and changing the baby appears to compound the problem. Thus, in some patients, carpal tunnel symptoms appear for the first time after the baby is born. In others, the symptoms may worsen. Incidentally, new mothers often develop tendinitis in the hands. This is also associated with extra use.

If you have pain or numbness in your hands, either when you're pregnant or after the baby is born, tell your doctor. These problems are usually simply treated, with a splint and perhaps a cortisone injection in the case of the carpal tunnel syndrome; with a splint, physical therapy, and occasionally a cortisone injection in the case of tendinitis. It isn't necessary to use medications, so don't keep your complaints to yourself because you are either pregnant or breast-feeding and don't want to take drugs. There are a lot of other things that can be done.

The following question is most often asked by women but is of obvious concern to men as well.

I don't want to have any more children. What type of birth control is best suited for someone with arthritis?

This is a question that must be decided by both partners in association with a physician. Whatever you decide on must be practical, as discussed below.

First, don't rely on the rhythm method. It's not very reliable.

If you have rheumatoid arthritis and your physician suggests birth control pills, it may be worthwhile to discuss this with a rheumatologist. Some arthritis specialists believe that birth control pills may result in flare-ups of the arthritis or cause other undesirable problems.

If the male partner uses a condom, the woman should also use contraceptive foam or jelly. The maneuvers required to put these, and a diaphragm, properly in place involve some dexterity, so be sure you can handle them comfortably.

Do not decide on a vasectomy or tubal ligation only because you are frustrated and depressed by your arthritis. These are difficult decisions that should be made when you are in a good frame of mind. If your arthritis is very active, the last thing on your mind may be having children. But once it is controlled you may feel quite differently.

My arthritis flares around the time of my menstrual period. Is that my imagination?

Probably not. In fact, this is a relatively common complaint. As frustrating as it may sound, there is little that can be done about this from a hormonal perspective. In other words, no one should try to manipulate your body hormones in order to make your arthritis better. On the other hand, it may be a good idea to increase your medication or perhaps get some extra physical therapy. Discuss this with your doctor.

14

Sports, Recreation, and Travel

My goal in treating people with arthritis is to allow them to lead as normal a life as possible. This includes participation in activities that are fun, such as sports, playing musical instruments, painting, and travel. Since these endeavors can present unique problems for a person with arthritis, they deserve special attention.

Sports mean different things to different people. For some they are an enjoyable way to keep in shape. For others the social factors predominate. For still others they represent challenges, sources of competition.

As mentioned in Chapter 8, Mickey Mantle was extremely disappointed when he could no longer play golf. I discussed this with Dr. Paul Greenberg of Dallas, Texas, Mantle's personal physician. "Here's a guy who played competitive sports since he was five," he said. "When he reached the point where he couldn't play golf, it really put him down." Once the former baseball player was treated, Dr.

329

Greenberg noted, "His whole life changed. He perked up all the way around."

Mickey Mantle's story reminds me of one of my own patients. Mary Baxter was 24 years old when she was diagnosed as having rheumatoid arthritis. Although she was doing quite well, her rheumatologist refused to allow her to participate in competitive sports. Sports probably mean as much to Mary as they do to Mickey Mantle. After competing in a number of women's sports in high school, she continued to play in various local leagues after graduation. In fact, when she discovered her town didn't have a women's basketball league she started one! The venture was so successful it soon expanded to a number of neighboring communities.

Predictably, Mary got depressed — not because of her arthritis, but because of her newly enforced lifestyle. It didn't take long after that for her arthritis to flare, and she sought another opinion. The second doctor became so fixated on her joints he forgot that the rest of her body and a mind were attached to them.

I was the third doctor Mary saw. When I first met her she really looked down in the dumps. She didn't smile during the interview or physical exam. Finally, when I told her my philosophy about treating patients with arthritis, she broke into a wide grin. I told her she needed physical therapy and would have to take one step at a time. Maybe she couldn't play basketball again, but at least she would get a chance to try. That was ten years ago. Mary has rarely missed a game or match since. Just like Lynn Adams, she has managed to remain competitive in sports despite the presence of rheumatoid arthritis.

I hope the following suggestions will allow you to continue to play your favorite sport as well as to keep traveling, whether for business or pleasure.

I love to play golf and hate to give it up because of arthritis. Do you have any suggestions for making the game physically less demanding?

Three of the people discussed in this book are avid golfers who have managed to continue the sport despite the development of arthritis. In addition to Mickey Mantle, Whitey Ford and Jack Kramer still play regularly. All three curtailed their golfing activities because of arthritis and were able to resume playing once they received appropriate medical care. All three play frequently, and Jack Kramer plays or practices an average of five days a week. You may be able to do as well. Don't forget to discuss your concerns with your physician, just as these gentlemen did. Make sure everything possible is being done to treat your arthritis.

Some modifications in your game may prove helpful as well.

• Use clubs with lightweight shafts and heads that are forgiving when you hit the ball off center.

• Experiment with different grips until you find one that is comfortable for you. Either build up the grips of your clubs or use air-cushioned grips. This makes gripping the club easier and absorbs more of the shock of hitting the ball.

• Use low-compression balls. They may not go as far but produce less shock when you hit the ball.

• Use a tee on the driving range. That way, if you miss, it is less likely your club will hit the ground and less likely you will hurt your arm from the impact.

• If you have to, use a cart. It's a lot better than not playing at all.

Do you have any hints that will allow me

to play tennis in spite of my arthritis?

Jack Kramer and Vic Seixas provided the following tennis pointers for people with arthritis.

• Warm up before playing. This should include stretching exercises and simulated shots, including ground strokes and service motion.

• Try to play on surfaces that allow you to slide before stopping. This puts less stress on your joints. Clay is ideal. As previously noted, Vic Seixas continues to play in tennis tournaments for players 65 and over and continues to be successful. Clay is his favorite surface, as it is less hard on his arthritic knees. Most of the tournaments he enters are week-long affairs, just as they are for younger players. He usually gets to the finals or semifinals. If the tournament is on clay, he usually feels fine by the end of the week. If it is on a hard surface he does not.

• Try using a racquet with a light head if you have arm trouble.

• Always keep warm. Start with a warm-up suit and take it off when you start to heat up.

• Tennis shoes should be well cushioned. Change shoes as soon as they show signs of wear.

• Be aware of your limitations. Vic Seixas jokes that he has been using two words with increasing frequency since he developed arthritis, namely "nice shot," as he allows his knees to rest while a difficult-to-reach ball passes by. If Jack Kramer's back acts up while playing, he stops and does a few stretching exercises. If the discomfort continues, he stops playing.

• Play with your joint problems in mind. For example, if you have trouble with an overhead slam, let the ball bounce and use a ground stroke. Norman Cousins loves tennis, but tendinitis and arthritis in his shoulder don't allow him to serve — so he serves underhand. At least he keeps playing.

Can I continue to go fishing even though I have arthritis?

Here are a few ways to make fishing easier and more comfortable.

• Since you'll be near the water, you will probably get wet. Make every effort to keep as dry as possible. Bring a towel with you and pay particular attention to drying your hands.

• Keep warm. Dress in a few layers, with the heaviest on the outside. Dispose of layers as needed.

• If you use rubber boots they will probably make your feet sweat. Wear a few layers of socks to insulate your feet and keep them as dry as possible.

• Use a reel with a large handle. It will be easier on your hands.

• Use a rod with a limber tip. It takes a lot of the effort out of casting.

• Suit your style of fishing to your physical needs. For example, bait fishing does not require as much casting as fishing with lures, and lures entail less effort than flies.

Individual sports such as jogging, bicycling, swimming, and skiing are marvelous ways to exercise. Be sure to discuss these sports with your doctor before participating.

I enjoy jogging but am afraid to continue because I'm afraid of getting arthritis. Should I stop?

There is little evidence to support the notion that jogging causes arthritis. However, the studies done so far have not been done over a long enough period of time to be conclusive. If you have had prior knee injuries, jogging may not be a good idea, especially if you experience pain or swelling after a run.

Being a Bostonian, it was only natural that I discuss running with Bill Rogers, a favorite son of Massachusetts. A world-class runner, this former Olympian held the American men's marathon record, which he set in 1975 while winning the Boston Marathon.

Here are a few of Bill Rogers' tips to make jogging safer and more comfortable.

• Buy comfortable jogging shoes that give you good support, especially in the arches. The heel should fit snugly, and the shoe should not be too stiff. Pay more attention to the fit than the brand.

• Joggers have a tendency to keep their favorite shoes too long. Once your shoes begin to wear, promptly buy another pair to help avoid foot, knee, and back problems. If you run on a slanted road, the outer sole will wear more quickly.

• The shoe insert usually wears before the

336

outer part of the shoe because of the pounding it takes. Replace the original inserts with a well-cushioned pair of your own as soon as this happens.

- Tie your shoes snugly but not tight enough to make them uncomfortable.

- Similarly, make sure your socks fit snugly and don't slide in your shoe. That is how you develop blisters.

- Dress appropriately for the weather. If you like to run in cold weather, purchase an all-weather suit. It will keep you warm and give you flexibility. Use mittens (they keep you warmer than gloves) and a hat.

- Run on a surface that has some give, such as grass or a track. Avoid running on pavement.

- If you run on a track and the rules allow, reverse direction halfway through your run to ease stress on the inside knee. Similarly, if running around curves hurts your knees, walk the curves and only run the straightaways. Be sure to check this with your doctor first, as he might not want you to run at all if you are experiencing discomfort.

- When you run, hit the ground with your heels and roll your foot forward.

- Relax your arms when you run. Swing them straight back and forth, not across your chest.

- Avoid hills. They significantly increase stress on your joints.

I asked Bill Rogers if he had any words of encouragement for would-be runners, and this is what he said: "Be smart and use common sense. Don't overdo it — it doesn't take that much to be fit. Everybody can be an athlete in their own way."

Any suggestions that will allow me to go biking without aggravating my arthritis?

- Be sure the bike, whether stationary or outdoors, is the right size for you. When seated with your leg in the lowest pedal position, there should be a fifteen- to twenty-degree bend at the knee.

- Pedal with the balls of your feet.

- Wear padded gloves. This reduces stress on your hands.

• Choose the right bike for you. Many people with arthritis prefer an upright touring bike to the racing style.

Do you have any suggestions regarding swimming and arthritis?

• Experiment with different strokes to find the right ones for you. It's often best to vary your strokes throughout your swim.

• Warm up by hanging onto the edge of the pool while kicking your legs through their range of motion. This loosens up your joints and muscles and increases blood circulation.

• If you are contemplating joining a health club to use an indoor pool, try it out first. Make sure the pool is not too crowded, so you can swim at your own pace. Also check out the water temperature. One of my patients recently left one health club to join another because the water was too cold.

• If you have neck problems, consider swimming with a snorkel when conditions allow.

• Use a kick board if you have shoulder or arm problems. This will allow you to exercise the rest of your body while protecting your upper extremities.

Will my arthritis prevent me from skiing?

Not necessarily, especially if you're willing to take a few precautions, as follows.

• If you're not exercising regularly, use your upcoming ski trip as a motivation to do so. Discuss the advisability of the trip as well as specific exercises with your doctor and physical therapist.

• Make sure your boots are comfortable and don't have any pressure points. If you can afford it, buy boots with built-in heaters.

• Use shorter skis than you're used to — it gives you more control.

• Don't use old-fashioned ski poles with leather bands that wrap around your wrists. They get caught easily and lead to injuries.

• Dress appropriately to avoid getting chilled. Use a number of layers so you can discard them if you get too warm.

• Avoid moguls and hard skiing. They put

tremendous pressure on your knees. Make wide, gentle turns.

• Be wary of poor snow conditions. Avoid ice at all costs.

• Waiting in long lift lines can stiffen you up and make you too hot or cold, depending on the weather conditions. Avoid them whenever possible, even if it means skiing an easier part of the mountain than you're used to.

• You may be confident in your own ability, but accidents are often caused by other people. Avoid areas where there are a lot of "hot dog" skiers.

• Don't push yourself. As with all activities, if your joints are uncomfortable — stop!

• If you're tired, don't go for that last run at the end of the day. That's when most accidents happen.

We now turn to the world of music and art.

I like to play the piano, but the arthritis in my hands is making it more and more difficult. Do you have any suggestions?

No one with arthritis should give up their favorite activities without a fight! Make it clear to your doctor that this is a real problem for you. You may be referred to occupational therapy and taught specific exercises to increase your dexterity and strengthen your muscles.

If you haven't seen a rheumatologist, consider a consultation. Strangely, arthritis may not be the cause of your problem. Musicians develop a number of specific problems, most of which are related to overuse of muscles and tendons.

The medical profession has become increasingly aware of the medical problems of musicians. In fact, a number of clinics devoted to these issues now exist. Most of these are located in major academic medical centers, so check to see if there is one in your city.

Finally, if all else fails, musicians can consider modifying their instruments. For example, a smaller electronic keyboard may provide a viable alternative to a standard piano.

Are there any ways painting can be made easier for the person with arthritis?

• Keep all painting supplies within easy reach and above waist level.

• Use brushes with large handles or build up thin-handled brushes with cushions or silly putty.

• Use a triangular rubber adapter if you are still having trouble handling the brush. They are usually used to build up pencil shafts, as previously mentioned, and can be found in school supply or stationery stores.

Any discussion of painting and arthritis would be incomplete without mention of Pierre Auguste Renoir, one of the most famous of the French Impressionist painters. Renoir was born in Limoges, France, in 1841. Interested in art from an early age, he attended an art academy in Paris where he came under the influence of a number of other greats of the art world, including Claude Monet. Success followed. Unfortunately, so did rheumatoid arthritis.

He suffered his first attack in 1897, the next a year later. Without the advantages of modern medicine, his illness got progressively worse. However, Renoir was an ingenious man, and he devised his own exercises. For example, he learned to juggle three small leather balls in order to keep his fingers limber. Despite his best efforts, his hands got progressively worse, as did the rest of his body, and he was soon confined to a wheelchair. At one point he partially regained his ability to walk, but it was such an enormous effort that he returned to his wheelchair. "I give up," he said. "It takes all my willpower. I would have nothing left for painting. If I must choose between walking and painting, I will take painting." Making that decision was like lifting a weight from his shoulders. His painting became more vibrant than ever.

His will was indomitable. As the arthritis got worse he continued to find ways to paint. Sometimes he gripped the brush with a wad of cloth. Other times it was strapped to his hands. He devised a series of rollers to which he attached his canvas. By turning a crank, the canvas could be positioned so that the area he was painting was always at a comfortable level.

Under these circumstances, he painted "Women Bathers," which hangs in the Louvre and which he considered his best work. He painted until the end. On the morning of the day of his death he worked for several hours on a still life with flowers. He died that night.

Renoir's pictures are full of life and color, joy and happiness. Some would say they are a marked contrast to a life devastated by rheumatoid arthritis. But were they? Some people refuse to be destroyed by negative events in their lives. Renoir was one of those people.

We now go on to an entirely different topic.

Travel can be very tiring. What can I do to make my trips as comfortable and uneventful as possible? First, do you have any suggestions to make packing easier?

• Use lightweight luggage. Don't lift it by its handle — use shoulder straps. Also, consider luggage with wheels.

• Always use porters or luggage carts when they are available.

• Bring an ample supply of dollar bills and change for tips. This will stand you in good stead throughout your trip.

• Pack as lightly as possible. Most people bring too much, so plan exactly what you will need.

Do you have any suggestions to make flying easier for the person with arthritis?

Air travel is generally the fastest form of transportation and is therefore usually the least arduous — especially after you get on the plane. The following can make your plane trip even less stressful.

• Find out whether fees are refundable, and if so, under what circumstances. This pertains to hotel accommodations as well as airline reservations. Consider trip cancellation insurance for peace of mind if you have any doubts.

• Take a nonstop flight if at all possible.

• If a nonstop flight is unavailable, be sure to leave ample time for making connections. Don't be misled by what seems like a reasonable amount of time. Many airports are not "passenger friendly." Distances between gates can be formidable. In some airports, changing terminals may mean taking a train or bus. Find this out ahead of time. Many airports provide motorized carts to help you get from one place to another — determine whether you'll need one of these beforehand. The airline or your travel agent can help you here. Be especially careful about allowing extra time for connecting flights during the colder months. If the original flight is delayed and the connecting flight leaves on time, your chances of making it are obviously diminished.

• If possible, travel during the week as opposed to weekends or holidays. It's less crowded (and often cheaper).

• Get your boarding pass ahead of time, either from your travel agent or from the airline through the mail. It saves waiting on lines, which are often endless. This way you will be able to go directly to the main gate.

• Use curbside check-in so you don't have to carry your bags. If taking a connecting flight, check your bags to the final destination so you won't have to worry about transporting them yourself.

• When making your reservations, ask about any special services you may require, such as special meals and ground transportation.

Do you have any suggestions regarding cars, trains, and ships?

• Car travel affords you flexibility, but some planning is necessary. Map out your route ahead of time. Make motel reservations in advance, or end your travel day relatively early. Don't wait until you are exhausted to start looking for a motel room. They fill up especially rapidly during the peak travel seasons, so don't take any chances.

• When renting a car, request power steering, brakes, windows, seats, and cruise control, all of which can make driving a lot more comfortable.

• If traveling by Amtrak, speak with someone at the "special service desk" about luggage transport, getting in and out of the train (there may be a few steps involved, and they will usually provide personnel to help you), obtaining a convenient seat accessible to dining and rest rooms, and anything else you have on your mind.

• Make similar requests of your cruise line if traveling by ship. In addition, obtain a cabin close to an elevator and a dining room seat close to the entrance if you have difficulty walking.

Are there special considerations when making hotel reservations?

• Request a room near elevators or within easy walking distance of specific amenities.

• It is helpful to stay in a hotel that provides airport transportation as well as transportation to local areas of interest.

• Be sure adequate room service is available. This is a real luxury on days when you're simply too tired to get to the dining room.

• Inquire about laundry facilities so you don't have to bring as much clothing.

Should I have any medical concerns when planning a trip?

• Discuss the advisability of the trip with your doctor. Do so as far in advance as possible, so appropriate lab tests, appointments, and therapy sessions can be arranged.

• Carry your medical information with you, including your diagnosis; a summary of your history; a list of all medications; your doctor's name, address, and telephone number; and similar information for a relative or friend who knows your history.

• If you have been or are on medications such as steroids, wear a Medic-Alert bracelet. This is also important if you have other medical problems such as diabetes, heart disease, or severe allergies.

• Ask your doctor what to do if problems arise during your trip. Specifically ask how to handle flares of your arthritis, side effects from your medication, and missed doses of medication. If you are going to a warm climate, ask about possible effects of the sun. Anti-inflammatory drugs and hydroxy-chloroquine can increase your sensitivity to the sun and cause a severe rash.

• Always carry your medications with you — don't put them in a bag being checked and don't leave them back in the hotel.

• Bring adequate medication for the trip as well as extra prescriptions.

• Since most medications used to treat arthritis must be taken with food, bring extra snacks.

• If going overseas, bring a doctor's statement regarding the medications you are taking. Not surprisingly, customs officials are often suspicious of vials of medication.

15

Using the Health Care System

The previous chapters were designed to increase your understanding of arthritic diseases and their treatment. It should be evident by now that a lot can be done for people with arthritis, including a lot they can do for themselves. You may already be seeing a physician who shares this philosophy. But what if you're not? What if you're not seeing a doctor at all? Or what if you are seeing someone who is generally interested in you and your disease, but you think there is room for improvement?

In exploring these and similar questions, this chapter will enable you to get the most out of the health care system. Remember, although there is a lot you can do to help yourself, you still need medical personnel to institute the appropriate treatment. No matter how enthusiastic you are, you still need help.

What can you do to guarantee your rights as a patient to the best possible care the medical profession can provide? And what are your responsibilities?

My arthritis is being treated by my family doctor and he doesn't seem particularly interested. In fact, when I told him my knees hurt, he told me his back hurt and there wasn't much that could be done for either of us. "After all, you're seventy-five," he said. He's in his mid-60s.

There are various red flags that indicate a second medical opinion is needed. If your doctor says you're too young to have arthritis and ignores your complaints, or that everyone gets it as they get older and there's nothing that can be done about it, see another doctor. Similarly, if your doctor liberally prescribes pain medication, especially drugs such as codeine, you should be concerned. Finally, if your physician has a one-dimensional approach — for example, prescribing medications to the exclusion of other types of treatment — you may not be getting the best possible care.

The person who asked the above question should definitely see another physician, but how does one go about this? Many patients feel uncomfortable questioning their doctor's authority; others are concerned about hurting their doctor's feelings. Either worry reflects badly upon the foundation of the doctor–patient relationship. Your health and well-being are your physician's primary concerns. Doctors should not feel threatened by any action that might improve your health.

So don't be shy — come right out with it. Remember, as a patient you are a consumer, a consumer of medical information and skills. As such you have certain rights, the foremost of which is that every one of your health concerns be appropriately addressed.

You can phrase your request for a second opinion in a variety of ways, but my advice is to *be honest*. Tell your doctor exactly how you feel. "Doctor, my arthritis is really getting me down. I'm frustrated. I can't do the things I want to do. Can you send me to a specialist for another opinion?"

You may be surprised at how supportive your doctor really is. He or she may not have truly realized the extent of your concerns, or may have been listening to you but not really hearing you.

On the other hand, the unfortunate reality is that some doctors are threatened by a request for a referral. Others are so poorly versed in this area of medicine that they are truly unaware of diagnostic and treatment considerations beyond their own relatively narrow purview.

Sarah Downer was 72 years old when she consulted me. A retired pharmacist, this bright, articulate woman asked her internist to refer her to a rheumatologist after a host of anti-inflammatory drugs not only failed to improve her osteoarthritis but also resulted in relatively severe heartburn. The next step was a pain reliever in the form of codeine, which she refused to take. She asked if there were any alternatives, to which her internist replied no, nothing further could be done. Refusing to accept his opinion, she insisted on the name of a rheumatologist, and my name was provided.

She was elated when I told her of additional therapeutic options, including splints and an exercise program. These treatments were quite successful. Mrs. Downer is more comfortable now than she has been in years — all because she had the gumption to ask her physician for a referral and refused to take no for an answer.

She continues to see her internist for her other medical problems — an indication of the soundness of their relationship. He is not angry with her, and she realizes that in the specialized medical world we live in, everyone can't know everything. However, she does wish he had been a bit more open-minded.

So don't hesitate to ask. Remember, *good doctors are not threatened by a request for another opinion*. In the example above, Mrs.

Downer's physician wasn't threatened, he was simply unaware of what a rheumatologist had to offer.

If my physician refers me to another doctor, or if I am seeking a physician to treat my arthritis, must I see a specialist?

Not necessarily, although the more complicated the case, the more you should consider seeing a rheumatologist. Family and general practitioners, internists, and orthopedic surgeons often take excellent care of their patients with arthritis, and from a mathematical perspective it is impossible for the relatively few rheumatologists in the United States to care for the thirty-seven million people with arthritis.

One hint: if your primary care doctor has made a number of attempts to treat you without significant improvement, you probably should see a specialist. For example, if your doctor thinks your knee pain is from arthritis, has treated you with a number of anti-inflammatory drugs, and you have not responded, the next step is to see a rheumatologist or perhaps an orthopedic surgeon.

Unfortunately, things don't always go according to plan. The next question is a logical extension of the above.

I asked my doctor for a referral but was told it wasn't necessary. What do I do now?

There are a number of ways to find a physician, one of the most obvious of which is to ask your friends and neighbors. Be specific when questioning them. Don't simply ask if they know a good doctor — ask if they know a good doctor who treats arthritis. First-hand accounts are particularly helpful in this regard. You can also call your local medical society, which probably maintains lists of specialists in various geographic areas of your state. A list of local rheumatologists is also available in the Yellow Pages. Look under "physicians" and then find the subheading "rheumatology." Be aware, however, that all the rheumatologists in a given area may not be listed. The listing is optional, and the busier specialists sometimes choose not to be listed.

Another option is to call local hospitals, most of which would be delighted to provide a list of specialists on their staffs. Similarly, if there is a medical school in your area, call and ask to be connected with the department of rheumatology. The secretary will provide you with a list of people in the department, and if you're friendly and honest about your needs, you may be surprised by how much information you can get. If there is a teaching hospital in your area (a hospital with interns, residents, and perhaps students), call and ask to speak with the chief medical resident. A chief resident has been on the staff long enough to know who are the good teachers and who keeps up with the medical literature. It may sound like an unusual approach, but it is often quite helpful.

You can call the local chapter of the Arthritis Foundation. If you have trouble locating a local chapter, write to the national office: Arthritis Foundation, P.O. Box 19000, Atlanta, GA 30326, or call 1-800-283-7800. You can also contact the American College of Rheumatology, 17 Executive Park Drive, NE, Suite 480, Atlanta, GA 30329, or call 404-633-3777.

Currently, there are only 2414 board-certified rheumatologists in the United States. The Arthritis Foundation and the American College of Rheumatology include physicians who are not board certified on their referral lists. However, both organizations use strict standards when formulating their lists. If it is important to you that the rheumatologist be certified, call his or her office to determine if this is the case.

Once you have a list of potential physicians, there are several ways to narrow it down. Start by trying to find a doctor who knows at least some of the doctors on the list. If you have had past experiences with a physician, call and ask for advice. If you're still seeing a doctor, even in an area unrelated to joint diseases, don't hesitate to ask. You'd be surprised by how much your gynecologist, your child's pediatrician, or even your dentist knows about the local rheumatologists and internists. If you have little or no access to physicians, ask friends or relatives to inquire of theirs. I am frequently asked for referrals by patients who are asking for third parties. Before making a final decision, call the prospective doctors' offices. Have a list of questions ready for the secretary — they are usually quite receptive.

Your questions should range from purely objective, practical issues to subjective concerns that are of particular concern to you. The former include fees, the amount of time allocated for initial and return appointments, the average amount of time you must wait for an appointment, willingness of the office to fit you in as unanticipated events occur, and the physician's phone accessibility.

Subjective concerns are quite different. Do you prefer a down-to-earth, friendly doctor or someone with a greater air of "professionalism"; someone who only explains a little or someone who explains a lot; someone who makes decisions about your treatment with you or someone who decides for you? Know your preferences — it is important that you find a doctor whose approaches suit you.

I want to be treated by the best doctor in the best medical center. How do I find them?

Some people have an obsession with finding "the best." What does that mean? There are no universal criteria by which rheumatologists and medical centers are judged, so it is impossible to declare who or which is the best. Physicians and medical centers get their reputations in different ways. One is by how much research they do and how much they publish. Although this assures us that particular individuals or institutions are up to date, at least in their area of expertise, it doesn't really tell much about how well they treat people. Find someone with whom you're comfortable. A great doctor for one person may not be good for another.

Once I am sent for another opinion, does that doctor take over my care?

Not necessarily. In some instances, especially if your problem is not overly complex, the consultant may send you back to your referring doctor with a list of suggestions. You may or may not need to see the consultant again, since your primary care doctor can certainly carry out these suggestions. Since the consultant will most likely specify the circumstances under which you should be referred again, this setup does not expose you to any undue risk, and it has certain inherent advantages. You probably feel more comfortable with your primary care doctor, who is more familiar with other medical problems you might have and whose care is probably less expensive. In rural areas, where specialists are not as accessible, this saves a great deal of travel as well.

The issue of travel is also germane for people willing to go great distances in order to get the "best" help. Not only is it unnecessary, it may be counterproductive. Since most cases of arthritis are chronic, it simplifies matters to have your care providers within a reasonable geographic area.

My rheumatologist thinks I need a hip replacement. How do I pick a surgeon?

A doctor sophisticated enough to think you probably need surgery will also provide you with a list of surgeons. Ask if your doctor has other patients who have been operated on by the various surgeons, and ask to speak with them. They may not be in a position to judge surgical skills, but you can determine if they were happy with the surgeon's attitude.

How can you determine the surgeon's skills? Without doing a statistical analysis, this is difficult, if not impossible. However, you can get a fair sense of a surgeon's experience and competence by finding out how often the surgeon performs the operation in question. If you need a hip replacement, for example, you are better off with a surgeon who does them as a matter of routine rather than infrequently.

Surgeons are an exception to the rule about getting your care close to home. If a surgeon with specific expertise is not locally available, don't settle for a nearby but inexperienced surgeon. If you live in an out-of-the-way area, there still may be a rheumatologist or two, or an internist with an interest in rheumatology, within relatively easy driving distance. On the other hand, although there may be a few orthopedic surgeons in the area, none may have experience with joint replacement. Under these circumstances you should be willing to travel a greater distance to get more sophisticated care.

Once I find my doctor, is there anything I can do to enhance my care?

In 1597 Francis Bacon wrote, "Knowledge is

power." When it comes to your care, nothing could be more true.

• Know your disease. Information supplied by the Arthritis Foundation indicates that thirty to fifty percent of patients with arthritis don't know the type they have. If you don't know your type, you probably do not understand the nuances of your illness. Also, in the event that other medical problems develop, it is very important for the treating physician, who may not be the one taking care of your arthritis, to be aware of the diagnosis. This is especially important for the less common arthritic diseases such as lupus.

• Ask your doctor about your medications. When you are placed on a new medication, be sure you know its name; why you are taking it; the dose; how it should be taken (for example, after meals, on an empty stomach); whether it interacts with other medications you are taking; whether it interacts with certain foods, alcohol, or additional medications you are not presently taking, especially over-the-counter medications; and its side effects and what to do about them.

I'm reminded of a middle-aged woman I saw in the emergency room when I was an intern. She complained of shortness of breath and heart palpitations. An EKG was taken, and her heart rhythm was indeed quite abnormal. The abnormality may or may not have been caused by specific medications. It was very important that this be determined, as it would influence her treatment.

When asked if she was on drugs she readily volunteered that she was. When I asked her the names and doses, she replied, "Two pink and one blue." Obviously this was of no help, but fortunately she remembered the name of her pharmacy. The correct information was soon obtained and it proved invaluable. What would have happened if she had not recalled the name of her pharmacy or was unable to communicate, or if it was the middle of the night and her pharmacy was closed? Her care would clearly have suffered. Don't just know the drugs you are on — keep a list of them on your person, and be sure another family member has a list as well.

• Review your medications with your physician at every visit. It is surprising how often discrepancies arise between the prescription and the way you're actually taking your drug.

• If you are seeing more than one doctor, inform each one of any changes another makes in your medication. For example, if your family doctor prescribes a new medication, be sure to remind him or her of your other drugs and to inform your rheumatologist of the new prescription.

• Whenever possible, obtain all medications in the same pharmacy. Pharmacies keep records of the medications their customers are taking, and frequently the pharmacist is the first person to spot a potential problem. Take advantage of your pharmacist's knowledge regarding side effects and drug interactions.

• Don't change your treatment program without consulting your doctor. Some patients stop taking medication, or at least reduce the dose, when they're doing well. The irony is that they may be doing well *because* they are taking their medication. On the other hand, some patients get discouraged if there is no obvious improvement within an arbitrary period of time. Yet anti-inflammatory drugs may take a few weeks to become effective. Remission-inducing agents may take months to work. So don't change your medication without discussing it with your doctor. An exception is the development of side effects (though your physician theoretically should have told you what to do under these circumstances at the time the medication was started).

• Ask your physician for appropriate reference material about your condition and its treatment. Your doctor may suggest you contact the Arthritis Foundation, which can supply you with the appropriate information.

• Put medical information you learn from the media into perspective. New research is aggressively reported by the press. Unfortunately, reports of new developments are often based on a single study, which may not stand the scrutiny of further investigation. Don't incorporate what you've learned on TV or in the newspaper into your treatment without calling your doctor.

• Plan ahead before your appointment. Jot down a few brief notes to be sure you ask about everything on your mind.

• Try to be as specific as possible when answering your physician's questions. I can't even count the number of times I've asked people where they hurt and they say, "Everywhere." Although patients with severe pain emanating from multiple areas may feel as if they are truly hurting everywhere, this is seldom the case. Describe the intensity of your pain and include the impact it is having on your life — for example, you may be having difficulty with keys or lifting pots.

• If there have been changes in your condition since your last visit, be sure to mention them — even if you don't think they are related to your arthritis or its treatment. Better yet, call your physician when the problem arises.

The following brief case history illustrates how important this is. Evelyn James is a 62-year-old woman with osteoarthritis who was being treated with ibuprofen. She was always fifteen to twenty minutes early for her appointments, so when she arrived almost a half hour late one day I was rather surprised. She told me she had just come from seeing an ear, nose, and throat specialist, whom she had consulted because of decreased hearing. As a matter of fact, it was the second such physician she had seen for this problem. Neither had offered an adequate explanation. I asked if she had told either physician that she was taking ibuprofen. She had not. I suggested she discontinue the ibuprofen, and within a short time her hearing returned to normal.

Decreased hearing is an unusual side effect that most anti-inflammatory drugs can cause. Mrs. James didn't consider the possibility of a causal relationship and therefore didn't tell me about the problem, nor did she tell the ear, nose, and throat doctors about the medication. Unfortunately, the two consultations cost hundreds of dollars — considerably more than the few cents it would have cost to phone me.

• Don't hesitate to discuss your personal life with your physician. If your arthritis flares after arguments with your spouse or if you're drinking more than usual because you're depressed, your doctor should know about it.

• If you don't understand your doctor's explanation or advice, say so and ask for clarification. If you still don't understand, don't be intimidated and *don't feel stupid!* Some physicians have difficulty explaining things clearly. That's not your fault, and since you didn't go to medical school you should not be expected to be familiar with medical jargon.

• If your doctor does not explain things, request an explanation — you are entitled to it. *Never blindly follow a doctor's orders without an explanation.* Remember, part of your physician's job is to be an educator.

• If you arrive home and realize you still have a question or have forgotten a piece of information, call back. Tell the secretary why you're calling — it will usually expedite a prompt response.

• Finally, and perhaps most important, always be honest with your physician. Discuss your concerns, no matter how trivial you think they are. If they concern you, by definition they are not trivial.

This point is graphically illustrated by Ronald Smythe, a 38-year-old patient of mine with rheumatoid arthritis. He was not doing as well as either of us would like, and I suggested he go on gold therapy. After hearing the pros and cons, he decided against the gold treatment. By the next visit he had gotten considerably worse. I again recommended gold, and he again refused. The very mention of the topic made him uncomfortable. I asked if he knew someone who had experienced side effects from gold, and he said he hadn't. I asked if any of the potential side effects were of particular concern, but they were not. He just didn't want to take the medication. I asked him to reconsider, and he reluctantly agreed. During the next visit I broached the subject one more time, and he appeared genuinely embarrassed. Realizing there was a hidden agenda, I finally cajoled him into the real explanation. He was having financial difficulties, and was afraid the gold would cost too much money — after all, gold is expensive.

I explained that there is indeed actual gold in the medication, but the amount is quite small and the cost in line with other similar medications. Relieved, he agreed to take the gold, had an excellent response, and we joked about the situation for years to come. We both learned our lessons. He agreed not to hide anything, and from that day on I've always told potential gold patients the cost of their therapy.

I'm satisfied with my doctor, but he can't always answer my questions. Can you suggest any other resources?

The Arthritis Foundation is an invaluable source of information. It is a national organization, and its mission is to find the cure for arthritis and to improve the quality of life for those affected by the disease. There are a number of local chapters throughout the country. Always start with the local branch. If it cannot be of assistance, contact the national office.

A partial list of services provided by the Arthritis Foundation follows.

• Referrals — As noted above, it can provide you with a list of physicians in your area interested in treating arthritis.

• Self-help courses — These courses increase participants' knowledge of their disease, improve self-care, and enforce the concept that people can help control their illnesses. They can be extremely valuable. Support groups are also available.

• Exercise classes — These include standard classes given at different levels as well as a water exercise program and a program for people with limited mobility.

• Information — The Arthritis Foundation publishes a large number of pamphlets covering a wide range of topics. They are available through your local chapter.

• Hot line — If you have questions, call your local chapter or the Arthritis Foundation toll-free number, 1-800-283-7800. A knowledgeable person will answer them or tell you how to find the correct answer.

• *Arthritis Today* — This is a bimonthly magazine available to members.

The Arthritis Foundation supports programs such as those described above as well as medical research. Money is needed to support these programs, so consider joining. By supporting the goals of the Arthritis Foundation you are helping yourself as well. Call or write your local chapter or the previously listed national numbers.

Another organization, the Ankylosing Spondylitis Association, publishes a quarterly bulletin and can provide you with material, including videotapes, about this illness. Write the ASA, P.O. Box 5872, Sherman Oaks, CA 91413, or call 1-800-777-8189 or 213-652-0609. They will also answer questions about spondylitis.

16

The Future

What does the future hold for you if you have arthritis? Will we ever be able to prevent it?

Before discussing the future, it's important to emphasize how far we have already come. The majority of patients with arthritis do well and are satisfied with their care. If your arthritis is not being treated, or you are unhappy with your treatment, do something about it! Speak with your physician or explore ways to change your care, as discussed in Chapter 15. You have to take advantage of the present before thinking about the future.

But the future certainly looks promising. New anti-inflammatory drugs are being developed that will probably be safer and more effective than those presently available. Medications that may be capable of healing cartilage are currently being tested. If successful, they will markedly decrease the number of people with osteoarthritis, or at least decrease the severity of the condition.

The more we learn about the causes of the various types of arthritis, the closer we come to curing and even preventing them. Rheumatoid arthritis and ankylosing spondylitis may be caused by microorganisms that attack genetically susceptible people. As scientists learn more about this process, they may be able to develop a vaccine to prevent it. The day may come when we vaccinate our children against the various types of arthritis just as we do against mumps, measles, and German measles.

Total joint replacements are invaluable for people whose joints have been destroyed by arthritis. As discussed in Chapter 9, this technology is being applied to more and more joints. The day will almost certainly come when any joint in the body can be replaced. Modern technology has already increased the life of these joints, and this will continue to improve.

The day will come when arthritis is a relic, merely a memory. It may not be in your lifetime, or mine, but it will happen. Until then, take advantage of everything modern medicine has to offer.

Index

Bursitis (cont.)
corticosteroids and, 172
physical therapy for, 187
ultrasound for, 191
x-rays of, 130, 133

Caffeine, 270
Calcimar, 182
Calcitonin, 182
Calcium, 241-243, 279
Calcium channel blockers, 182
Callahan, Kevin, 19, 22-23
Cancer, 112, 117, 122, 179
Canes (walking sticks), 197, 273-274
Capsules (anatomy), 29
Carafate, 170-171
Carbohydrates, 246
Cardiac disease, 68, 194, 241, 297
Carpal tunnel syndrome,
91-93, 172, 325-326
Cars, 220-221
Cartilage, 29, 30, 130, 134
Causes of arthritis, 60-81
CBC, 115-117
Cementless joint replacement, 231
Cervical traction, 195
Charisse, Cyd, 32
Chemical laboratory tests, 117-119
Children, bearing of. *See* Pregnancy
Chiropractic, 280-283

Diagnosis (cont.)
  Physical examination; Symptoms

Isometric exercises, 201

THORNDIKE PRESS hopes you have enjoyed this Large Print book. All our Large Print titles are designed for easy reading, and all our books are made to last. Other Thorndike Large Print books are available at your library, through selected bookstores, or directly from the publisher. For more information about current and upcoming titles, please call or mail your name and address to:

THORNDIKE PRESS
PO Box 159
Thorndike, Maine 04986
800/223-6121
207/948-2962